# Understanding Existential Health for Dementia Care

*Understanding Existential Health for Dementia Care* is a groundbreaking book that describes how existential health can enrich and expand bio-psycho-social approaches to dementia care, recognizing that well-being extends beyond physical, neurological, and cognitive symptoms. This book equips professionals, clinicians, and caregivers to integrate existential dimensions into person-centered care, emphasizing the role of meaning in life and emotional connection for dealing with illness and suffering.

Beginning with an introduction to the concept of existential health, the book connects this to an overall understanding of health related to dementia care. Core themes include the coincidence of suffering and meaning, fear of dementia, challenges to personhood, and multicultural perspectives. The book then provides an overview of how existential health can enhance person-centered care, addressing different types of dementia, neurological changes, emotional factors, and daily life functioning. The final section provides examples of existential support, including tools for meaningful conversations and existential exploration. The last chapter weaves together the book's thematic threads, highlighting how past experiences contribute to present sense of meaning, identity, and connectedness in people with dementia.

It is valuable reading for professionals in dementia care—nurses, psychologists, doctors, and chaplains—as well as for caregivers seeking inspiration and students in medicine, nursing, psychology, theology, and social work.

**Lars Johan Danbolt** is Head of Research at Research Center for Existential Health, Innlandet Hospital Trust, Norway, and adjunct professor at MF Norwegian School of Theology, Religion, and Society, Oslo, Norway. Main research fields are existential health, clinical psychology of religion, and practical theology.

**Tatjana Schnell** is Professor of Existential Psychology at MF Norwegian School of Theology, Religion, and Society, Oslo, Norway, and Fellow at the Humanistic University Berlin, Germany. As head of the Existential Psychology

Lab, she focuses on fundamental questions of how to conceptualize and measure meaning in life and on the nexus of meaning in life and health, work, worldview, suffering and dying, civic engagement, and alienation.

**Gry Stålsett** is a specialist in Clinical Psychology and Associate Professor of Psychology of Religion at MF Norwegian School of Theology, Religion, and Society, Oslo. She serves as the Head of Clinical Practice at Bispehagen, Center for Existential Therapy and Counseling in Stavanger, Norway.

**Peter la Cour,** PhD, is health psychologist and adjunct professor at MF Norwegian School of Theology, Religion, and Society, Oslo, Norway. Main research interests are existential health, the psychology of pain and suffering, and psychology of religion.

# Understanding Existential Health for Dementia Care

**Edited by
Lars Johan Danbolt, Tatjana Schnell,
Gry Stålsett and Peter la Cour**

Routledge
Taylor & Francis Group

LONDON AND NEW YORK

Designed cover image: Getty Images via Rawpixel

First published 2025
by Routledge
4 Park Square, Milton Park, Abingdon, Oxon OX14 4RN

and by Routledge
605 Third Avenue, New York, NY 10158

*Routledge is an imprint of the Taylor & Francis Group, an informa business*

© 2025 selection and editorial matter, Lars Johan Danbolt, Tatjana Schnell, Gry Stålsett and Peter la Cour; individual chapters, the contributors

The right of Lars Johan Danbolt, Tatjana Schnell, Gry Stålsett and Peter la Cour to be identified as the authors of the editorial material, and of the authors for their individual chapters, has been asserted in accordance with sections77 and 78 of the Copyright, Designs and Patents Act 1988.

*British Library Cataloguing-in-Publication Data*
A catalogue record for this book is available from the British Library

ISBN: 9781032853468 (hbk)
ISBN: 9781032829425 (pbk)
ISBN: 9781003517733 (ebk)

DOI: 10.4324/9781003517733

Typeset in Times New Roman
by codeMantra

# Contents

# Contributors

**Sverre Bergh** is a specialist in psychiatry and Head of research at Research Center for Age-related Functional Decline and Disease, Norway. His main research interest is in dementia, old age psychiatry, and healthcare service.

**Önver A. Cetrez** is Professor in Psychology of Religion and Cultural Psychology, Uppsala University. He studies migrants and refugees with attention to ethnic and religious identities, resilience, coping, existential health, acculturation, and conflict.

**Knut Engedal** is a retired professor of geriatric psychiatry at the University of Oslo, Norway. His main interest in research is about dementia diagnostics, treatment, and care.

**Ingvild Hjorth Feiring** is a PhD candidate at the Research Center for Age-related Functional Decline and Disease, Norway. Her main research areas are dementia and nursing home practices.

**Knut Hestad** is professor emeritus of neuropsychology at the Norwegian University of Science and Technology, Trondheim, and researcher at Innlandet Hospital Trust. His main interests in research are dementia, HIV/AIDS, and biological determinants for mental disorders.

**Bendik Sparre Hovet** is a psychology and philosophy student at the University of Oslo. In an internship with Tatjana Schnell, he has explored the SoMe Card Method in existential conversations with patients in a nursing home.

**Tor-Arne Isene** is hospital chaplain at the Department of Mental Health Care, Innlandet Hospital Trust, Norway, and researcher in the Research Center for Existential Health at the same hospital. His main research interest is existential health in dementia care.

**Peter Kevern** is Professor of Values in Health and Social Care at the University of Staffordshire, UK, where his research and teaching focus is on the overlap between religion and dementia.

**Bjørn Lichtwarck**, MD, PhD, is Senior Researcher and Chief Physician in the Old Age Psychiatry Department at The Innlandet Hospital Trust, Norway. His main research interests are dementia, medication, and person-centered care.

**Lars Lien** is a specialist in psychiatry and public health. He is professor in public mental health at Inland University, Norway, and current president of the Norwegian Psychiatric Association.

**Silje Mathea Nylund** is psychologist and has done research in existential dementia care affiliated with The Research Center for Existential Health, Norway.

**Shahram Shaygani** is a specialist in psychiatry, an addiction medicine specialist, a psychoanalyst, and a psychotherapy supervisor. He is a board member of the Norwegian Psychiatric Association and works as a clinical chief physician at the Trasopp Clinic in Oslo, Norway.

**Sturla J. Stålsett** is Professor of Society, Religion and Diaconal Studies at MF Norwegian School of Theology, Religion, and Society, Oslo, Norway. His research interests include liberation theology, social justice, and religious plurality. He is also a rock musician and singer-songwriter.

**Hans Stifoss-Hanssen** is professor emeritus at VID Specialized University, Oslo. His main research areas are related to existential health, ritual practices, diaconia, and pastoral care.

**Trine M. Struer-Tranberg** is psychologist, with special interest in social psychology, existential psychology, and palliative care. She is currently working in the public mental health sector in Denmark.

# Editorial introduction

*Lars Johan Danbolt, Tatjana Schnell,
Gry Stålsett, and Peter la Cour*

## Existential health in the care for people living with dementia

Why do we need a book like this?

We see three main reasons: First, existential health is increasingly gaining attention in healthcare services, especially concerning dementia and other late-life conditions. Second, there is still limited knowledge about what existential health entails and its significance for treatment and care. And third, dementia profoundly threatens an individual's sense of meaning in life, identity, and connectedness, core aspects of existential health. This makes a book like this both timely and necessary.

Existential health is on the political agenda. Recently, the Swedish government highlighted existential health together with an overall understanding of health. However, there are various approaches to understanding what existential health is. In this book, we link existential health to four key aspects: it involves subjective *experiences of the self*; it is connected to *systems of orientation* in life; it includes the experience of a *meaningful life*; and it is *expressed to others* through opinions and attitudes, as well as feelings and body language.

Dementia touches the core of an individual's identity and relationships with others. This means that existential health care must, of course, provide the best possible physical and medical support, but also go beyond the bio-psycho-social aspects to assist individuals in their efforts for maintaining a sense of significance, coherence, orientation, and belonging, which form the content of the experience of life as meaningful.

Dementia often causes people to lose parts of their autobiographical memory, which makes it difficult for them to hold onto a coherent sense of who they are. However, their identity does not necessarily disappear; rather, it often becomes more relationally dependent. Life stories, fragments of personal history, and narratives that help individuals make sense of their experiences remain important, even as the ability to express these stories may diminish.

In dementia care, those affected, their families, and healthcare providers often experience existential distress, reflecting struggles with identity and connectedness when familiar structures dissolve. Addressing these concerns requires a compassionate framework that validates and expresses emotions, enabling moments of genuine connection and alleviating existential distress. Through shared understanding, people living with dementia may find a renewed sense of connection and meaning, despite the challenges posed by cognitive decline.

*Understanding Existential Health for Dementia Care* can contribute to person-centered approaches and enhance the quality of reminiscence therapy, storytelling, or by means of other approaches help bridge the gap between past and present, fostering meaning in life and reinforcing the individual's identity and sense of connectedness.

For many people, existential health relates to ways of understanding life's challenges, and for providing comfort and hope. Cultural traditions, rituals, familiar artifacts, music, and art can help maintain a sense of normalcy, connecting individuals to their past and helping them find meaning in the present.

In dementia care, supporting existential health involves recognizing the complexity of human experience, including the paradoxes of suffering and meaning. By understanding existential health, caregivers can help individuals with dementia maintain dignity, identity, and connectedness, even in the face of cognitive decline. This approach not only enhances the quality of care but also affirms each individual's inherent worth, regardless of cognitive ability. Additionally, integrating existential health into person-centered care can deepen caregivers' sense of purpose, enriching their work with greater meaning.

This book explores existential health in relation to biological, psychological, and social health, examining its role in a holistic understanding of overall well-being. We also discuss the intersection of existential health with current knowledge about dementia and its place in person-centered treatment and care.

The book has three parts:

- *Part I* covers existential health in dementia care, examining the coincidence of suffering and meaning, fear of dementia, challenges to personhood, multicultural considerations, and examples from existential person-centered care.
- *Part II* looks at how existential health can strengthen person-centered care, detailing types of dementia, brain changes, the daily impact of dementia, and the role of emotions and life stories.
- *Part III* provides examples of existential support, including methods for conversation, clinical exploration, and the use of online peer forum for

care providers, and concludes with a summary chapter that discusses how past experiences can be present and contribute to a sense of identity and connectedness for people living with dementia.

A key message from this book is that existential health is not solely an individual experience but also a collective one that happens in community, in nursing homes, and other places where people with dementia live their lives. This means that existential health is also a matter of fostering existentially healthy care environments.

# Part I

# Existential health, suffering, personhood, and culture

# 1 Existential health and persons with dementia

*Peter la Cour*

In the process of dementia, something gradually disappears, and something changes. It can be described as a loss of nerve cells in neuroscience and a loss of cognitive functions in neuropsychology, and changes in character can be described in personality psychology, social psychology, or sociology. But through all the changes in the person with dementia, one thing remains unchanged, that is, the presence of a subject within, a subject who is experiencing living a life, who is being present in our shared world, and who has some sense of continuity, of being the same. The living subject within the person with dementia *exists* and has the capacity to alternate between states of well-being and states of suffering. This is existential health. We have no better word for it.

Existential health is a term under development, and there have been several suggestions to give it content and more clarity, as will be seen later. However, both the words existential and health can seem fluffy when we think more deeply about them. That is true for many things we just take for granted. As the quote attributed to Saint Augustine says, when we do not think about *time*, we know exactly what it is, but as soon as we think about it, we do not know what it is. The same goes for both the term health and the term existential. The aim of this chapter is to go deeper into our concepts of health, especially existential health and to relate them to the process of dementia.

## Health

There is no fixed definition of health, which makes it very difficult to deal with in science, where clear definitions are a must because they are essential to determine whether something is the case or not the case. The word health itself might be scientifically meaningless without a specification of what is meant in the specific case. Nevertheless, the word has an intuitive meaning for all of us.

The problem of a good definition of health was present when the World Health Organization (WHO) was established in 1946. The WHO was founded to improve health in the whole world, but what aspects of health should it

DOI: 10.4324/9781003517733-2

look after? Was it hunger? Lack of happiness? Absence of hospital systems? Soon after its establishment, the WHO came out with this proposed definition of health (World Health Organization [WHO], 1948): "Health is a state of complete physical, mental and social well-being and not merely the absence of disease or infirmity."

There are two important elements in this definition: The word *well-being* and the identification of three areas in which well-being can unfold: *physical, mental, and social*, these three areas, no more, no less. The naming of the three was repeated much later in 1977 when G. Engel announced his proposal for an integrated model of health, the Biopsychosocial Model (Engel, 1977), suggesting that health was an integration of the three areas and that all three areas are always present in every aspect of health. What is the problem here?

## Existence

The problem is the missing subject. What is missing is the person who is *experiencing* the well-being – and if well-being is absent, then the person who is experiencing suffering is missing; the person who is living a life that can be affected by physical, mental, and social illnesses. In that way, if a person is physically well, mentally well-functioning, and has a good social network, but still feels that the life is not worth living, feels unhappy, or worthless – this person will be considered in good health according to the definitions.

What kind of life is worth living? Who can be the judge of that but the only person who actually lives it? It is the personal evaluation of the life lived and felt that can lead to existential well-being. In that sense, existential well-being may be the most important kind of health of all; without the sense of a life worth living, all the other areas are inferior. This very essential issue is completely missing from the WHO definition of health.

This is not a new thought or critique. There have been several attempts to include existential experience in the definition of health within the WHO. In 1984, there was a proposal to add the term spiritual to the list of physical, mental, and social, but the proposal failed after much discussion because people could not agree on what the term spiritual meant. Different people had very divergent perceptions of it (Peng-Keller et al., 2022). The same critique has been raised toward the biopsychosocial model, where there is also no subject, the person experiencing the sickness is simply not present in the model (Álvarez et al., 2012). But it is the sick, subjective person it is all about, because it is the sick person who can suffer to a degree that life is valued as not worth living, and who can decide to commit suicide. On the contrary, it is the sick, subjective person who can choose to live as intensely as ever despite serious illness. Caring for that subject – also called the humanistic perspective in medicine – is also absent in the usual health definition. Something essential is missing.

It is not because the category of subjective existence is empty of words; we have lots of content-loaded terms and words concerning exactly this, dating back to the beginning of humanity. Let us recapitulate some of the most important qualities in life: Meaning in life, purpose, dreams, appreciation of art, sense of significance, hope and optimism, life thirst, belonging somewhere, longing, striving, and acceptance. We can even talk about acceptance of death. We can talk about a full life, when a life has been lived with contentment, and there is a sense of the days being full – who would not want that in the end? We also have names for all the opposites: Meaninglessness, purposelessness, visionlessness, gloom, feeling isolated, hopelessness, pessimism, feeling homeless, without any goal, life discomfort, no ability to accept, ever holding on to what has been.

All these words are not really taken seriously in modern mainstream cognitive psychology, which is based on principles of learning. To look for an unfolding and expansion of the words, one has to look to the humanistic disciplines, such as philosophy, theology, literature, and art. In psychology, one has to look to *humanistic psychology* to put flesh on the bones and also to the subsection called existential psychology, which is specifically devoted to such aspects of life.

Existential philosophy and existential psychology can get quite mixed up, and it is sometimes difficult to tell the difference, but existential philosophy has the longest history and this way of thinking of life has always been a branch of any theologian tradition – it is the question of what human existence is all about. As a unique discipline, existential philosophy includes names such as Kierkegaard, Heidegger, Satre, and Camus, and all these put the emphasis on the inner life of the subject, the experience of life seen from within. However, there has been very little new material developed in the last half-century (Cooper, 2003; Flynn, 2006).

Existential psychology has taken over to some extent, and it is usually intertwined with some sort kind of psychotherapeutic practice, beginning with Dasein-analysis (psychiatrists Binswanger and Boss from 1920 onwards), further developed by names such as Viktor Frankl (logotherapy), Rollo May, Irvin Yalom, and Emmy van Deurzen Smith (existential psychotherapy). These thinkers see human life as a challenge and seek to help their clients meet that challenge in a fruitful way. Some of these theorists speak about existential givens (basic polarities in human life that need to be confronted) and of the method of phenomenology as the main way to have any knowledge of another person.

## The spontaneous reality

Unfortunately, both existential philosophy and existential psychology seem very academic and hard to reach for people with no education in that kind of thing. They seem to be far away from the everyday experience of existential matters and reflections on what life is for ourselves and for others, and from our own immediate and constant experience of the bodily condition and the presence of well-being or suffering. Such experiences are *private* but very *basic*. We can share some of them with others in conversation or show some of them in behavior, but they are basically not shared in full; no one can feel exactly what it is to be in another body or the intensity of another person's suffering or how it is experienced to live with dementia.

Yet we assume that this kind of consciousness of being existent is also present even in the final stages of dementia. It is the hallmark of being *awake*, not asleep, or unconscious. There is an experience of life, well-being, or suffering in there, although the personality around it may have changed during dementia.

The spontaneous experience of living is the first and basic component of existential health.

## The orientation system

An important part of well-being is the sense of meaning. Meaning in life is a central concept in both existential philosophy and psychology. It was the main concept for Viktor Frankl, and in the later years it has been further explored in empirical ways by several. Psychologist T. Schnell has made significant contributions unfolding that meaning comes from something different from person to person. She calls such personal meaning creators *sources of meaning*, and she points out that in psychology we do not speak about the meaning *of* life, but the meaning *in* life (Schnell, 2021).

Sources of meaning are part of a person's orientation system, the system of subjective evaluations of what has worth and importance in life and what is considered less important. It is this system of attitudes and beliefs, which are subjective, private, and often even unconscious, and it cannot be shared with anybody in full. In the orientation system also lies the ability of acceptance. The ability to accept suffering and death may be two very essential elements for well-being in dementia.

The orientation system is another basic component of existential health.

## Qualities and expressions

The orientation system can give rise to qualities such as, for example, having a purpose in life, belonging somewhere, being optimistic, feeling guilt and shame, or feeling inner homeostasis. Some of these qualities are actually visible to others, who can recognize these qualities as characteristics of the other, maybe as the essence or nature of this specific individual. The orientation system can also give rise to qualities such as self-confidence and a sense of significance, and it can result in what is called quality of life, a term with several attempts to be captured and measured empirically in questionnaires. It has been debated how successful these attempts have been to actually assess the quality of life, because which questions should be included and which questions should be excluded as markers? Is quality the same for a busy young person and a person living with dementia? The doubts and debates are rooted in the fact that the existential is fundamentally subjective and therefore not able to be shared and measured in full.

The life orientation system and the existential qualities can also have outward expressions in more coarse and visible forms such as religious beliefs or political views, and they can be noted by others in expressions such as choice of lifestyle, or in some personality traits.

Existential qualities and expressions are also components of existential health.

## Dimensions of health

It has now been argued that the existential is fundamental, natural, spontaneous, and, in some ways, the most important dimension of life. Existential health can be sensed in terms of well-being – precisely the main word in the WHO 1946 definition of what health is – and its opposite: suffering. So existential health is basically the well-being of the subject, and it can move between the states of existential well-being and existential suffering.

Two other components were also mentioned: The orientation system (meaning) and the expressions/qualities of the existential. It would be nice to go further and continue with a consistent, and one-dimensional definition and further description of what existential health is. But that would be asking too much, as none of the other dimensions of health mentioned (biopsychosocial) can fulfil such criteria. They are all heterogeneous, multiple, and atomized, when taking a closer look. They are all palettes with very different colors and textures on them and with no clear borders to be found.

What is physical health and disease? It has been divided into hundreds of specialities that even may not know much of each other. There is not much in common between the disciplines of, for example, neurosurgery, occupational medicine, and the speciality of nutrition.

The same is certainly true of mental health – no one has ever agreed on a definition, but several attempts to define "psychological health" have been made by different psychological schools and ideologies. Again, there is not much in common between, for example, mental health diagnostics, organizational psychology, and the field of existential psychotherapy.

Social health is mentioned authoritatively by WHO, but it is perhaps the least defined of the three. What is bad social health? We do not even have such a term in our language. Once more, there is not much in common between the work in occupational medicine, the building of socially beneficial urban areas, and the expertise of anti-smoking campaigns.

So, of course, we have to acknowledge that the dimension of existential health will also be multifaceted, complex, and of a non-uniform nature. The WHO has reconsidered their definition of health several times, and in 1984, an important, completely new thought emerged (WHO, 1984). It came from the perspective of health promotion, and it took health away from the individualized view of well-being. WHO here claimed that health is...

the extent to which an individual or group is able to realise aspirations and satisfy needs and to change or cope with the environment. Health is a resource for everyday life, not the objective of living; it is a positive concept, emphasising social and personal resources, as well as physical capacities.

The key word here is not well-being, but *resource*. Health is not seen as well-being but as a resource for living and unfolding aspirations. With this definition, health actually embraces suffering, at least to some extent, and the associations with this definition of health might lead in completely other directions.

If health is seen as a personal or group resource, the next question will be: A resource for what? The answer is "for everyday life," a very broad term most probably simply meaning "life." Again, we are left with rather philosophical concerns, but this time perhaps evolutionary theory can be of help in setting relationships between the different dimensions of health.

First, the environment can have or lack the resources for creating and maintaining life. This makes sense even from the very first expression of life on Earth, and it still makes sense to talk about environmental health (for example, in terms of the availability of food and non-toxic air to breath). The next basis for creation of life is the social component, as life for all complex species requires some form of reproductive meeting of egg and sperm, and for us humans, our life requires social surroundings (moms, dads) to take care of children for at least five to ten years. In this way, environmental and social resources (health) can be seen as the most basic kind of health, and if they are not functioning, life itself must cease.

But if it is healthy, environmental and social health are resources that make a living body possible, whether it is just a single cell or a human. When the living body is healthy, it functions as a resource to make something higher possible: the learning system, the mental capacities that we call the psychological apparatus. When the mental (psychological) is healthy, it can serve as a basis for a new level, which we can call the existential, the consciousness of being a living being and the orientations in the world.

In this way, the combination of principles of *emergence* (a higher level emerges from a lower level with new qualities not present in or deductible from the lower level) can rank the dimensions of health and also give the dimensions of health a direction, a purpose for well-functioning. The purpose is not to demand perfect health on every level, but the levels to be *healthy enough* to serve and maintain the next level. Also in this way, existential health can be perceived as the most valuable kind of health to obtain.

## Existential health – toward an integrated understanding

Existential health is a currently evolving concept. One of the first proponents was psychologist Valerie DeMarinis (DeMarinis, 2008) closely followed by Cecilia Melder (Melder, 2012). They linked existential health tight to the subjective orientation system. Other developments have focused on subjectivity and the concept of suffering (Binder, 2022), and a Norwegian group (Nygaard et al., 2022) has made an integrative proposal for a definition with more than one component.

In accordance with this line of thinking, it is here suggested that existential health must include at least four main groups of components: (1) A basic group of components that is purely experiential, the first-person perspectives of experiences. (2) A group of life orientation system components, basic assumptions, and world view. (3) A group of existential qualities such as quality of life and meaning in life. (4) A group of existential expressions in which the existential components will be partially visible to others, some even measurable such as happiness and life philosophy.

## The social nature of existential health in dementia

Of these groups of components, the basic subjectivity, the experience of living a life might be of most relevance in dementia and dementia care.

Some existential philosophers claim it as a "given" that humans are fundamentally existentially isolated. Humans are existentially alone because the subjective experience is never fully shared with others (Yalom, 1980), we are born alone and die alone (Breitbart, 2017).

One could very easily argue the opposite: We are not born alone; we are born as a result of the meeting and mating of two parents, and we are born physically as close as is ever possible to our mother – and mostly also surrounded by other committed people like the father or grandmother. We are usually happily welcomed into a family that will selfishly maintain our life throughout childhood. If this is not the case, the baby will die. Without the others, we are dead.

We do not die alone either because we die full of experiences, memories, and relationships with others, or we die with a vocabulary of insights and words invented and developed by the collective of humanity. Without words and language, we are not human; we have no instrument to develop a human consciousness of the world. It is understandable what some existentialists mean when they say that the subject is never fully accessible from the outside, but both biologically and humanistically human beings are deeply embedded in each other, the social, the group, and the environment, as other existentialists emphasize.

This deep social rooting might play a special role in dementia. It is often said that dementia is more a disease of the relatives than of the person suffering from dementia. If we think in terms of health-as-function this may make some sense, because dementia represents the slow cancellation of the function of the cognitive abilities. The well-functioning of the psychological faculties makes the existential dimension possible, and when the psychological function disappears, the existential has no grounding any longer.

Perhaps most importantly, the human tendency to worry and speculate, which is always on the move, seems to disappear when dementia progresses, whereas it is fully active in the relatives, who care for optimizing the life surroundings for the demented person, food and drink supplies, relationships with others and the quality of life, the proximity and acceptance of death – all such worries, speculations, anxiety, loss, and suffering.

Especially in the final stages of dementia, when speech is no longer possible and there is no sign of recognition of the carer or family member, suffering does no longer seem to be recognizable in the demented person, maybe besides physical pain. Are people with terminal dementia lonely? Do they think of and relate to death? Do they feel and identify as the same person as they always have, although everything has changed? We simply do not know, we must rely on our own immediate sense of what goes on.

But carers and relatives, as fundamentally social beings, will still relate to and experience well-being and suffering in relation to the demented person and will provide the necessary life-sustaining elements. We relate and have memories and history with the demented person because we as humans are born social in groups that care and worry for each other. Doing so is meaningful and serves our own existential health well.

## References

Álvarez, A. S., Pagani, M., & Meucci, P. (2012). The clinical application of the biopsychosocial model in mental health: A research critique. *American Journal of Physical Medicine and Rehabilitation, 91*(13 Suppl.1), 173–180. https://doi.org/10.1097/PHM.0b013e31823d54be

Binder, P. E. (2022). Suffering a healthy life—On the existential dimension of health. *Frontiers in Psychology, 13*, 77. https://www.frontiersin.org/journals/psychology/articles/10.3389/fpsyg.2022.803792/full

Breitbart, W. (2017). Existential isolation. *Palliative and Supportive Care, 15*(4), 403–404. https://doi.org/10.1017/S1478951517000621

Cooper, M. (2003). *Existential therapies*. London: Sage.

DeMarinis, V. (2008). The impact of postmodernization on existential health in Sweden: Psychology of religion's function in existential public health analysis. *Archive for the Psychology of Religion/Archiv Fur Religionspychologie, 30*(1), 57–74.

Engel, G. L. (1977). The need for a new medical model: A challenge for biomedicine. *Science, 196*(4286), 129–136. https://www.ncbi.nlm.nih.gov/pubmed/847460

Flynn, T. (2006). *Existentialism: A very short introduction.* Oxford: Oxford University Press. https://doi.org/10.1093/ACTRADE/9780192804280.001.0001

Melder, C. (2012). The epidemiology of lost meaning: A study in the psychology of religion and existential public health. *Scripta Instituti Donneriani Aboensis,* 2012. https://journal.fi/scripta/article/view/67417

Nygaard, M. R., Austad, A., Sørensen, T., Synnes, O., & McSherry, W. (2022). 'Existential' in *Scandinavian Healthcare Journals*: An analysis of the concept and implications for future research. *Religions, 13*(10). https://doi.org/10.3390/rel13100979

Peng-Keller, S., Winiger, F., & Rauch, R. (2022). *The spirit of global health : The World Health Organization and the "spiritual dimension" of health, 1946–2021.* Oxford University Press. https://global.oup.com/academic/product/the-spirit-of-global-health-9780192865502

Schnell, T. (2021). *The psychology of meaning in life.* London and New York: Routledge.

World Health Organization (WHO) (1948). Preamble to the constitution of the World Health Organization as adopted by the International Health Conference. *Official Records of the World Health Organization.* https://cir.nii.ac.jp/crid/1571135650541969152

World Health Organization (WHO) (1984). *Health promotion: A discussion document on the concept and principles: Summary report of the Working Group on Concept and Principles of Health Promotion,* Copenhagen, 9–13 July 1984 (p. 8). Copenhagen : WHO Regional Office for Europe. https://iris.who.int/handle/10665/107835

Yalom, I. D. (1980). *Existential psychotherapy.* New York: Basic Books.

# 2 Dementia as an existential challenge

## Acknowledging the paradox of suffering and meaning

*Tatjana Schnell*

Accepting a dementia diagnosis is a profound challenge, as the disease fundamentally alters life trajectories. This struggle is well-documented among those diagnosed with dementia and their caregivers (Yates et al., 2021). The difficulty of acceptance extends beyond patients and loved ones; even healthcare professionals who specialize in dementia care find it particularly challenging to help patients and families come to terms with the diagnosis (Gwernan-Jones et al., 2020). This chapter discusses the existential challenges associated with dementia and the possibility of developing an encouraging perspective through acknowledging our existence's contradictory nature.

## Paradoxes of existence

As humans, we often grapple with the opposites of existence. We celebrate life while ignoring its finite nature, seek joy and happiness while overlooking the value of negative emotions, and strive for strength while forgetting that strength also lies in embracing vulnerability.

In the 15th century, Nicholas of Cusa, an early Christian proponent of humanism, introduced the concept of *coincidentia oppositorum*, the coincidence of opposites. He suggested that seemingly contradictory principles – such as finitude and infinity, light and dark, good and evil – are not only reconcilable, but that they are ultimately interdependent.

This approach to reality is reflected in various later philosophies. Søren Kierkegaard addressed the tensions between freedom and necessity, faith and reason, and despair and fulfilment. Martin Heidegger described how existential anxiety opens the door to an authentic life. Theologian Paul Tillich explained the necessity of the "courage to despair" – a term contradictory in itself.

It may seem paradoxical to reconcile these opposites, yet life cannot be understood without death, nor can joy be appreciated without knowing sorrow. Indeed, it is not the easy and pleasant life stories that are associated with higher mental health, well-being, and maturity. As McAdams and McLean report (2013), these qualities develop when people have experienced suffering

DOI: 10.4324/9781003517733-3

and adversity and can meaningfully integrate these experiences into their life story. Other psychological approaches support this conclusion. Confronting the negative, rather than avoiding it, doesn't imply a pessimistic outlook on life, as one might expect. Instead, it has been shown, for instance, with regard to the acceptance of death, to be associated with lower anxiety (Spitzenstätter & Schnell, 2022) and improved quality of life (Brabbins et al., 2023). Proactively engaging with distress may seem inappropriate or absurd at first, especially in a challenging situation such as dementia, yet it helps us see, and live, our humanity more clearly.

## Dementia as an existential challenge

A dementia diagnosis interrupts lives. So-called positive illusions are shattered: We realize we don't have everything under control, suffering isn't only experienced by those who "deserve" it, and things don't always take a turn to the better. A dementia disease can be understood as a *boundary situation*, as described by philosopher Karl Jaspers (1954). Its occurrence is not a mistake that can be avoided, a problem that can be solved, or a misunderstanding that can be clarified. It is a condition that we have to deal with when it arises.

Boundary situations confront us with the limits of our rational understanding. They pertain to experiences of inevitable suffering, mortality, uncertainty, guilt, and struggle. Jaspers identifies three responses to boundary situations:

1 Derailment, leaving us paralyzed and ready to give up.
2 Suppression or denial, attempting to manage challenges through superficial solutions.
3 Acceptance, which embraces doubts and contradictions, ultimately making us stronger.

This third approach, which acknowledges our vulnerability, illustrates the coincidence of opposites. Strength is rooted in accepting weakness. Just as we know light because we know darkness, resilience arises from facing vulnerability. This broader view of life applies to dementia too, not only for individuals and relatives but also in the professional realm. For healthcare workers, adopting this existential perspective adds a meaningful dimension to their work, benefiting both themselves and those in their care.

## Supporting existential health in dementia

Dementia impairs cognitive functioning and our understanding of identity. It challenges self-images as autonomous agents and competent problem-solvers. In line with the biopsychosocial model of health, we can and should view these processes from medical, psychological, and social perspectives. Yet, an important aspect is missing if we remain at these levels only. It is the perspective of what it *means* to be in this situation: to the person who is going to live with dementia, to relatives and friends, to caregivers. Even with proper medication, a robust psyche, and supportive relationships, dementia, like many other diseases, confronts us with the fragility of health and mind, the inevitability of suffering, of losing oneself and each other.

Acknowledging this is difficult. Even in critical situations, humans can suppress the obvious. This is evident in hospice visits when relatives declare, "You'll be better soon!" or during hospital calls reduced to conversations about the weather. It also occurs in doctor-patient interactions where attempts to address existential experiences are redirected to the biomedical realm (Larsen et al., 2022). By excluding the existential dimension, we obscure our view of existential health. Beyond biological, psychological, and social aspects, health requires an existential foundation.

## Meaning in life as an existential foundation

An existential foundation provides a vantage point from which to approach critical life events. It arises when people trust in their lives' meaningfulness, based on experiences of significance, orientation, coherence, and belonging. These experiences are not necessarily conscious. They are based on more or less implicit and intuitive evaluation processes concerning our being in the world – in relation to ourselves, to others, and to our environment. Experiencing myself as mattering, as oriented, coherent, and belonging is more, or something else, than what the biopsychosocial model of health calls for, i.e. being symptom-free, mentally healthy, and socially supported. Existential experiences retain their validity even in the face of their opposites: Significance meets nonsense; orientation alternates with loss of control; coherence emerges from flux, and belonging ultimately leads back to being myself. Existential health, in this sense, is a preparedness to accept these paradoxes of existence. Only a realistic view of what is painful, meaningless, or burdensome allows us to deal with it appropriately. It is a first step toward acknowledging that life is worth living even in modes other than strength and efficient functioning, and that a meaningful life is not jeopardized by facing the human condition.

## Suffering as an inevitable part of life

Suffering is an inescapable aspect of the human condition – physically, emotionally, and existentially. Acknowledging this does not mean glorifying pain and suffering but taking an honest, realistic view of the world. Whereas suffering can become detached from its causes and persist beyond them, we can also detect valid reasons for suffering.

Physical pain signals bodily malfunctions or external dangers, and it is crucial for taking appropriate measures. This becomes evident in rare conditions like CIPA (Congenital Insensitivity to Pain with Anhidrosis), where insensitivity to pain puts affected individuals at great risk. Chronic pain, however, lacks such a function and requires different treatments and approaches.

Emotionally, suffering can express dysfunctional psychological processes manifesting in depression, anxiety, or personality disorders, for instance. Yet emotional suffering can also be appropriate. In many cases, suffering experiences are constructive and necessary for maintaining mental health, including fear, worry, grief, guilt, shame, and anger. They indicate danger, caution, missing someone or something dear, making mistakes or crossing boundaries, or that something is going wrong and requires opposition.

Existentially, suffering can arise from fear of death, now considered a transdiagnostic construct underlying various mental disorders. It also comes from a sense of existential isolation, a subjective feeling of fundamental separation from the world and others, that one's worldview is not understood or shared. Additionally, there can be anxiety about the immense freedom in shaping our lives, what Kierkegaard called the "dizziness of freedom." Multi-option paralysis can result – an inability to decide given the multitude of possibilities and their consequences. People also suffer from experiences of meaninglessness – of life itself or their own lives.

Existential suffering is characterized by the inevitability of many of its causes. Mortality, freedom, and absurdity are features of the human condition that cannot be prevented. While it is possible to ignore them to some extent, confronting them, however painful, seems important and necessary to clarify our self- and world-understanding and appropriately address challenges (Schnell, 2022).

In relation to dementia, accepting suffering as part of human life can be expressed in an attitude like this: I don't have to fight the fact of the disease. I can accept that it has occurred. Although this acceptance is initially painful, it is a good prerequisite for perceiving, understanding, and appropriately dealing with the situation – whether as an affected person, a relative, or a professional.

Such an attitude can be supported in the care and treatment of people living with dementia. This requires *existential communication*, touching on fundamental questions of what it means to be human: Who am I – without memory, without orientation in the present or future? How will I remain myself, preserve my dignity? How will I remain a partner, father, mother? These are fears about autonomy, security, and remaining a meaningful member of society.

Health personnel should address these fears proactively. In many cases, patients are afraid of not being taken seriously in these matters. With good reason, as studies show: attempts to communicate existential questions or fears are often ignored by staff (Larsen et al., 2022).

This can even be the case when care and treatment are based on the approach of person-centered care. A review and synthesis of qualitative studies (Gwernan-Jones et al., 2020) concludes that person-centered care is considered the method of choice in the context of dementia. Nevertheless, hospital staff often experience that the prevailing care culture prioritizes certain tasks, routines, and physical health, thus undermining person-centered care.

Moreover, this very approach can *prevent* existential issues from coming to the forefront. In a study by Andersen and colleagues (2020), physicians reported that all their patients had existential concerns, but the physicians usually did not address them. They felt not sufficiently trained for this, felt it was too private, or that it contradicted their treatment approach. This was even the case if they followed a patient-centered care approach, which emphasizes shared decision-making, a symmetrical relationship between patient and health personnel, and patient responsibility. As a consequence, existential issues are not tackled if patients – or their relatives – do not insist on it. This, in turn, requires sufficient awareness, courage, and ability on their part. Indeed, many patients experience this as an obstacle (Andersen et al., 2023). They report that medical aspects are prioritized at the expense of existential concerns, and that this affects both their treatment and well-being. It is therefore practically necessary that health professionals signal their willingness to listen to and take existential concerns seriously.

## The subjective nature of suffering

People perceive critical events differently. Suffering is subjective. What is a manageable loss for one person is a tragedy for another. Different symptoms of dementia have different meanings for those affected. The person-centered care approach can take this into account. In addition, environmental and contextual factors have significant effects on how burdensome something is perceived to be, and there are many ways to modulate experiences of suffering:

Negative sensations are amplified when we attend to them, focus our attention on them. This is necessary sometimes; at others, it is not. It is helpful to understand this as an option: We can consciously decide to pay attention to negative sensations. Likewise, we can decide to direct attention to something else – ideally, to a meaningful activity.

If we are able to consciously allow negative sensations, to proactively address them instead of waiting for them to come to the fore, they lose part of their frightening character. And the lower the fear of pain or negativity, the less burdensome it is experienced (Rogers & Farris, 2022). By contrast, the more we fear pain, symptoms, or limitations, the more we focus on them, expect them, and the more they burden us.

Learning experiences also play a crucial role in what we fear or perceive as distressing. We acquire knowledge not only through direct experiences but also by observing the actions of others. In the context of dementia, it is therefore vital to carefully consider the information we disseminate and how we convey it. Communication should be balanced, presenting both critical aspects and examples of successful coping strategies. This approach is particularly important because research has shown that general anxiety and a sense of loss of control can intensify the perception of pain and suffering. Consequently, also products, services, and environments such as homes, nursing facilities, and hospitals should be designed to instill a sense of security, comfort, and stimulation. This thoughtful approach can significantly enhance the ability of individuals to cope with the challenges posed by dementia (Rodgers, 2022).

## Meaningfulness as a motivator and a buffer

Meaning in life influences our mental and physical health, even our lifespan. This happens both through the motivational function of life's meaning, and because of its buffering function (cf., Schnell, 2021). When we see a meaning in our life, we find it worth living. This motivates to act accordingly: to invest time and energy into health behaviour, take preventive measures, eat healthily, exercise sufficiently, take care of hygiene, stick to health protocols, etc. Such behavior is not always pleasant, often time-consuming, and sometimes burdensome. A sense that life is meaningful and worth living is a crucial motivator to commit to health behavior nonetheless.

Moreover, meaningfulness serves as a buffer between stressors and distress (cf., Schnell, 2021). Having a sense of coherence, purpose, significance, and belonging creates a foundation for facing critical events, and it acts as a shield, or buffer, reducing the impact of stressors and enhancing resilience.

The four elements of meaningfulness can be supported in all life situations, also when living with dementia. Caregivers' knowledge of the sources of meaning of a person living with dementia helps to shape activities and surroundings in such a way that they are perceived as *coherent* and offer *purposeful* engagement. References to what people have done in their lives and how they have left their mark enable experiences of *significance*. The existential experience of *belonging* can be supported by social inclusion, but also by the very concrete design of one's personal "place in the world," of one's dwelling (Heidegger); through touch – e.g. by body-centered therapy or in contact with animals, or through experiences of being connected to a larger whole, whether through participation in religious or spiritual rituals, or through the experience of nature (Han et al., 2016; Isene et al., 2022).

## Conclusion

An existential perspective on life emphasizes the importance of acknowledging the paradoxes of existence. While suffering is an inevitable part of life, it is also a deeply subjective experience that we can actively engage with.

This engagement is supported by an existential foundation, grounded in the trust that life can be meaningful – even in illness. At the onset of dementia, adopting this perspective can aid those affected to confront the illness and recognize it as part of life.

Knowledge of personally relevant sources of meaning enables carers – both relatives and professionals – to ensure that individuals living with dementia continue to experience orientation, significance, coherence, and belonging, and thus maintain a sense of meaningfulness, even as their agency declines.

Lastly, these considerations also apply to carers themselves. Maintaining a balance of personal sources of meaning is crucial to nurture their own existential health.

## Literature

Andersen, A. H., Assing Hvidt, E., Hvidt, N. C., & Roessler, K. K. (2020). 'Maybe we are losing sight of the human dimension'–physicians' approaches to existential, spiritual, and religious needs among patients with chronic pain or multiple sclerosis. A qualitative interview-study. *Health Psychology and Behavioral Medicine, 8*(1), 248–269.

Andersen, A. H., Illes, Z., & Roessler, K. K. (2023). Regaining autonomy in a holding environment: Patients' perspectives on the existential communication with physicians when suffering from a severe, chronic illness: A qualitative Nordic study. *Journal of Religion and Health, 62*(4), 2375–2390.

Brabbins, L., Moghaddam, N., & Dawson, D. (2023). Accepting the unacceptable? Exploring how acceptance relates to quality of life and death anxiety in a cancer population. Emerald Open Research, *1*(2). https://doi.org/10.1108/EOR-02-2023-0003

Gwernan-Jones, R., Abbott, R., Lourida, I., Rogers, M., Green, C., Ball, S.,..., & Thompson Coon, J. O. (2020). The experiences of hospital staff who provide care for people living with dementia: A systematic review and synthesis of qualitative studies. *International Journal of Older People Nursing, 15*(4), e12325.

Han, A., Radel, J., McDowd, J. M., & Sabata, D. (2016). Perspectives of people with dementia about meaningful activities: A synthesis. *American Journal of Alzheimer's Disease & Other Dementias, 31*(2), 115–123.

Isene, T. A., Thygesen, H., Danbolt, L. J., & Stifoss-Hanssen, H. (2022). Embodied meaning-making in the experiences and behaviours of persons with dementia. *Dementia, 21*(2), 442–456.

Jaspers, K. (1954). Psychologie der Weltanschauung. Berlin, Göttingen, Heidelberg: Springer.

Larsen, B. H., Lundeby, T., Gulbrandsen, P., Førde, R., & Gerwing, J. (2022). Physicians' responses to advanced cancer patients' existential concerns: A video-based analysis. *Patient Education and Counseling, 105*(10), 3062–3070.

McAdams, D. P., & McLean, K. C. (2013). Narrative identity. *Current Directions in Psychological Science, 22*(3), 233–238.

Rodgers, P. A. (Ed.). (2022). *Design for People Living with Dementia.* London: Routledge, Taylor & Francis Group.

Rogers, A. H., & Farris, S. G. (2022). A meta-analysis of the associations of elements of the fear-avoidance model of chronic pain with negative affect, depression, anxiety, pain-related disability and pain intensity. *European Journal of Pain, 26*(8), 1611–1635.

Schnell, T. (2021). *The Psychology of Meaning in Life*. London: Routledge.

Schnell, T. (2022). Suffering as meaningful choice. An existential approach. In A. Austad & L. J. Danbolt (Eds.), *Ta vare. En bok om diakoni, sjelesorg og eksistensiell helse* (pp. 3–14). Oslo: VID.

Spitzenstätter, D., & Schnell, T. (2022). The existential dimension of the pandemic: Death attitudes, personal worldview, and coronavirus anxiety. *Death Studies, 46*(5), 1031–1041.

Yates, J., Stanyon, M., Samra, R., & Clare, L. (2021). Challenges in disclosing and receiving a diagnosis of dementia: A systematic review of practice from the perspectives of people with dementia, carers, and healthcare professionals. *International Psychogeriatrics, 33*(11), 1161–1192.

# 3 The fear of dementia and the challenge to personhood

## Exploring the depths of our existential dread

*Peter Kevern*

"Mum first died on the 12th of May 2019
When she couldn't work out how to prepare her legendary roast anymore.
The style icon of the Covington estate,
Mum died as a fashionista the day she couldn't get dressed into her colourful outfits …
She died as the Queen of Christmas
When she refused to have dinner with the family.
She died again when she asked me,
her son, what my name was.
She died as Dad's Rock,
After 52 years of marriage,
The day she looked straight through him.
On 10th March 2024,
Mum died a final time,
Surrounded by her family".
*With dementia, you don't just die once, you die again, and again, and again.*
(Alzheimer's Society, 2024b)

When in March 2024 the Alzheimer's Society (the UK's largest and most influential dementia charity) released this advert on television, radio and social media, it was to a flurry of debate and bafflement. Responses recorded as comments under the YouTube video of the advert were bewilderingly diverse, but almost uniformly impassioned. For some, this was a crass and insensitive representation of dementia that frightened those recently diagnosed or caring for somebody living with the condition; that undid years of messaging about the possibility and necessity of 'living well' with dementia; and that neglected the many ways in which (in their experience) loved ones continued to 'be themselves' despite the losses and deficits. For others, the advert was no more than an honest, unflinching look at the brutal reality of loving somebody disappearing before their eyes, dissolving under the onslaught of a condition David Keck memorably called, "Deconstruction Incarnate" (Keck, 1996).

DOI: 10.4324/9781003517733-4

This capacity of dementia to inspire a sort of existential dread almost certainly explains the deep fear that it inspires in Western societies. It is consistently emerging as the most feared disease of all among older people in the UK, USA and Australia (Alzheimer's Research UK, 2021). It is my belief that, if we seek to understand what existential health means for people living with dementia we must understand the existential challenge that it poses, not just to them but to all of us. Because the dread of dementia is itself a source of existential suffering for the person who lives with dementia, and the fears we share as a society deeply affect the ways in which we respond to them.

In this chapter, I will explore the features of this dread – what drives it, what feeds it – by reflecting on some of the key messages hidden in the short passage with which I opened the chapter. I will then point to ways in which scholars, practitioners and people living with dementia themselves have resisted the 'deconstruction' embedded in the encounter with dementia and sought to meaningfully reconstruct personhood in the face of the condition.

## Delving deeper – hypercognitive society

*Mum first died on the 12th of May 2019*
*When she couldn't work out how to prepare her legendary roast anymore.*

If we dread dementia because it rouses our existential fear of death itself, then in order to understand the existential needs of people who live with dementia we need to examine what we think is dying. As Bryden says, "...Dementia is often thought of as death by small steps, but we must ask ourselves what is really dying..." (Bryden, 2005, 159). If I fear that dementia will rob me of whatever 'makes me myself', then we may want to examine our assumptions about what that is.

The classic answer is that what is dying is the 'inner self', the 'true identity' who thinks, feels, acts and remembers in an inner space which needs to be maintained and protected. There are two dimensions here: we imagine that each of us has a 'true self' that exists independently of everybody else in an inner space; and that we know about this 'true self' because it performs mental actions in the abstract, apart from the world around us. This understanding of what makes me myself is embedded in a long tradition of Western thinking about the nature of the person, beginning perhaps with Rene Descartes' famous formula, *Cogito ergo sum* – "I think, therefore I am": my very being is to be found in my capacity to think, and from that develops my self-consciousness, my capacity for intentional action and my interactions with the world around me.

The upshot is that, without consciously intending to, we have found ourselves in a 'hypercognitive' society, in which "the image of human fulfilment is framed by cognition and productivity" (Post, 2002, 34). We understand ourselves as a bundle of shifting functions and roles held together by an isolated inner self that reflects, chooses and moulds the coherent narrative that comprises our personhood, the thread of continuity that persists over the course of our life. Dementia strikes at the heart of what we consider to be ourselves: our ability to think coherently, to find a 'truth' at our centre, from which we can 'be ourselves' in whatever we do in a shifting world. It follows that we will have nothing to offer to support the existential well-being of a person living with dementia if we believe their rational mind is where their personhood resides: for the cognitive faculties are indeed disappearing, inexorably and inevitably. We need to find a different way of seeing. In the words of Jesus Christ, "Do not be afraid of those who kill the body but cannot kill the soul. Rather, be afraid of the one who can destroy both soul and body in hell" (Matt 10.28 NIV). If our 'soul' is our cognitive self and its narrative, it is no surprise that we are afraid of dementia. But, as we can already see in the case of Descartes, constructs of identity depend on philosophy and social context (Post, 2002). How might rethinking the personhood of the person living with dementia in their social network cast light on the question of who we really are?

## The social self

*She died as the Queen of Christmas*
*When she refused to have dinner with the family.*

Examining the passage with which this chapter opened, we can see that there are two senses to the statement that 'Mum died' while she was still physically alive. On the surface, it seems to be about 'Mum's' individual subjectivity, the inner spark that makes her herself. However, on closer examination we can see that most of the references to dying are to 'social death', to the ways in which social connections and other people's understanding of her as a person are being lost.

Discussions of existential health tend to revolve around a concept of the person as an independent maker of meaning, creating their self-narrative in isolation. But there is a substantial sociological tradition that stresses the importance of social connections in this process. In the phraseology of African Ubuntu philosophy, "I am because we are". We may even say that the 'inner self' that I think I am is not my own property but only 'lent' to me by the community surrounding me.

When thinking of the personhood of somebody living with dementia, the existential importance of this social dimension has long been recognised. More than 30 years ago, Stephen Sabat pointed out in his seminal paper that the 'I' is a complex construct, encompassing two distinct senses of self: Self 1 (personal identity) and Self 2, comprising all the 'selves' we are in relation to others (Sabat & Harrej, 1992), and as my cognitive capacity diminishes through age or dementia, it will be the community's respect and memories of me that will maintain me as an individual. Responsibility for "conscious, collective authorship of the self-narrative" (Radden & Fordyce, 2006) will pass increasingly from me to those around me, and with it my existential integrity.

This means that the existential well-being of a person living with dementia may be more vulnerable to the actions and reactions of others around them than would be the case for most adults. There is the danger of what Tom Kitwood refers to as 'malignant social psychology': the mechanism by which our unreflective assumptions and poorly handled attempts to 'help' may end up alienating and disempowering the very person we want to support (Kitwood, 1997).

This implies that 'social death' may be more than a metaphor for the way in which somebody becomes absent from the social circle. By ceasing to recognise the personhood of the person with dementia in the midst of the social circle, perhaps their very existence is being erased as their 'self-narrative' dies of neglect? In this way, is it indeed possible to die "again, and again, and again"? If so, it follows that the way we recognise this person cannot be separated from the way we talk about them, and their existential health may ultimately depend partly on our social discourse. This brings us to the question of language: how do we talk about persons, and how do we talk about how dementia affects them?

## Talking of dementia and the person as the 'living dead'

*With dementia, you don't just die once, you die again, and again, and again.*

The choice of language in the advert we are examining matters, because it 'positions' the person with dementia in a particular way that can influence their existential well-being. Our medicalised language is of warfare, of mind-robbers, attacks and strikes by an alien invader (George, 2010); and the metaphor of the 'zombie', as someone whose personhood has departed leaving behind an animated body of decaying flesh that refuses to die, has been deployed in popular media discourse around dementia. A similar range of metaphors is commonplace across literature, film and news media (Low & Purwaningrum, 2020).

It is possible to interpret this curious use of dehumanising language as expressive of our relentless search for imagery that will grab our attention and monetise it; but it also has a political and intentional aspect. Thus, in her defence of the language of 'dying again, and again, and again' in the advert, the CEO of the Alzheimer's Society points to its potential to force the hand of policymakers: "Every time we shy away from talking about it, we give policy makers and decision-makers cover to ignore dementia and take action on something else" (Alzheimer's Society, 2024a). Similarly, Megan-Jane

Johnstone has argued from her deep dive into the Australian media environment that the use of a narrative of invasion, injury, loss and dehumanisation about dementia both fuels and is driven by the debate on Assisted Dying (Johnstone, 2016). Our discourse on meaning, purpose and value is one in which existential anxiety about dementia is only one of the forces competing for our attention and to shape the language world in which we move.

It is not easy to treat someone as a person with full dignity if the label 'zombie' has been attached to them. It is almost impossible to contribute to the "conscious, collective authorship of the self-narrative" if the narrative is of invasion or 'hollowing out' of the person. In general, then, it seems very likely that the language that we develop to express our fears and to 'cope with' the progress of dementia in ourselves and others actually 'locks us in' to that way of thinking, ultimately amplifying our fears while closing off other ways of thinking that may open up new hope.

> Part of our moral challenge in adapting to ageing populations is about semantic choice… Specifically, our societal perspective might be less distressing if individuals and their families could see dementia not just as a "loss of self", but as a change in self not so unlike many others a person undergoes in other life stages.
>
> (George, 2010, 587)

For this reason, campaigners for the well-being of people living with dementia have, for several decades, paid close attention to the language in circulation and consciously worked to develop more positive imagery – hence, my use in this chapter of the term 'person living with dementia' rather than 'dementia sufferer' or 'dementia victim', terms which bracket off personhood and from the start.

## *Not* dying 'again and again and again'

This analysis of the advert has laid bare some of the dimensions of the experience of dementia represented by "dying again, and again, and again" and so helps to point us to some of the essential features of existential care. In the remainder of the chapter, I will retrace our steps and discuss briefly some of the responses to the existential challenge of dementia.

At the level of the **language and rhetoric** around dementia, many carers and support workers have made conscious efforts to shift the language from the impersonal to the personal, and from the passive to the active. The language used has shifted over the last 40 years from references to, collectively 'the demented' (who appear to have no personhood at all) to 'demented people' (who have personhood, but are defined primarily by their condition) to 'people living with dementia' (who are not only persons, but active agents who are not circumscribed by their dementia). As well as consciously counteracting the depersonalised, non-agentic 'zombie' language prevalent in popular discourse, this shift in terminology restores the person, their agency and their needs to the front and centre of the conversation and so lays the groundwork for sustained attention to their existential needs. Existential care begins with the language that is used, both in reference and in conversation: the discourse must change.

At the level of the **social self**, there is a growing recognition within the field of dementia care generally that to care for and recognise the person entails caring for their social self: their networks and the memories, the roles and narratives embedded in them. As the person's individual ability to maintain their self-narrative becomes compromised by loss of focus, agency and operative memory, and as capacity to communicate may be impaired, so the contribution of those around them becomes more fundamental. Welcoming social networks such as the European Meeting Centres programme and the Church of England's Dementia Friendly Churches initiatives can support the people living with dementia both directly by providing social support, and indirectly by 'caring for the carers' so that the person's closest associates can continue with the "active, collective authorship of the self-narrative". As the person's dementia progresses and communication becomes more difficult, John Swinton stresses the importance of developing communities of attentiveness as the presupposition for supporting existential health (Swinton, 2017); and even in the later stages of the condition, Julie Simpson's impressive PhD work has shown how a detailed and 'ethnographic' involvement with the individual, their community and history, can enable sensitive and fruitful responses to their existential needs (Simpson, 2024).

At the level of the **personal, centred self**, there is an attempt by some people living with dementia and those close to them to tell a different story of the individual from the narrative of loss and repeated 'dyings', by valuing aspects of personhood that are less cognitively or socially determined, and finding existential meaning in attributes such as faith, forgiveness or contemplation (Horsburgh, 2024). The examples we have of people who have found a form of existential well-being in and through their experience of dementia vary very widely in the resources they use and the answers they arrive at. Three well-known examples may help to make this point.

First, there is Christine Bryden, who I referred to earlier in this chapter. She was a senior civil servant in the Australian government when she started to display the first symptoms of dementia; now, some 25 years on, she continues to write and speak on the subject. By virtue of this unusual trajectory, she brings to her account of the experience her advanced communicative ability and her extended reflection on the meaning of what is happening to her:

> ...Dementia is often thought of as death by small steps, but we must ask ourselves what is really dying. Hasn't the person with dementia reached that place of "now," of existing actively in the present?

I believe that people with dementia are making an important journey from cognition, through emotion, into spirit. I've begun to realise what really remains throughout this journey is what is really important, and what disappears is what is not important. I think that if society could appreciate this, then people with dementia would be respected and treasured.

(Bryden, 2005, 159)

If for Bryden the way to existential well-being was via a letting-go and active living in the present, for Wendy Mitchell the response was almost the opposite. She used her considerable organisational and planning skills (honed as a non-clinical manager in the NHS) to compensate for the growing deficits and to maintain control over her life for more than ten years, chronicling her progress in three books (two of which so far have been best sellers). Her control extended to her choice of death, by voluntarily ceasing to eat or drink at what she considered the right time. In her final blog she wrote:

Dementia is a cruel disease that plays tricks on your very existence. I've always been a glass half full person, trying to turn the negatives of life around and creating positives, because that's how I cope. Well I suppose dementia was the ultimate challenge... Yes, dementia is a bummer, but oh what a life I've had playing games with this adversary of mine to try and stay one step ahead... I didn't want dementia to take me into the later stages; that stage where I'm reliant on others for my daily needs; others deciding for me ... The Wendy that was didn't want to be the Wendy dementia will dictate for me.

(Mitchell, 2024)

Finally, Jennifer Bute treats her dementia not as a problem to be solved but "an unexpected gift, a wonderful opportunity and great privilege" (Bute, 2022). She sees it as an opportunity to contribute something distinctive and valuable to others by combining her medical knowledge as a GP with her insights within the framework of her encompassing faith. She is comfortable with the concept that the God in whom she believes ordained for her to have dementia and has devoted her energies to speaking, generating resources, running groups and writing a book in order to help different communities of people to understand how to respond to people with a lived experience of dementia.

In each of these cases, the existential well-being of the person living with dementia has been secured by resisting the narrative of incremental death that structures the Alzheimer's Society advert, along with its looming threats of social death, loss of agency and 'zombification'. While each is explicitly aware of their approaching physical death, they find meaning within that horizon in distinct ways, creatively reframing their experience and expanding their social networks even as some capacities are being lost.

In summary, in this chapter I have argued that we need to respond to our fear by reframing what dementia means for us, and what it means for the people living with the condition. When we treat people living with dementia as 'zombies', as socially isolated, or even as already dead, we are failing in our duty to care for their existential needs. But we are also failing to care for our own needs. To overcome our fear, we need to see how somebody living with dementia continues to be a human being even if they have changed; and to challenge the assumptions and imagery that separate us from them.

## Questions for reflection

Do you fear what will happen to you if you have dementia? If so, what aspect of it do you most fear?

Have you ever come across somebody (in experience or through reading) who seems to be 'living well' with dementia? If so, what was their secret?

Governments and pharmaceutical companies are investing large sums to look for a cure for dementia. How could that money be used instead to improve the existential well-being of people who are living with dementia now?

## References

Alzheimer's Research UK. (2021). *Dementia attitudes monitor wave 2.* Cambridge: Alzheimer's Research UK.

Alzheimer's Society. (2024a). *Alzheimer's Society CEO responds to criticism of their latest TV campaign.* https://www.alzheimers.org.uk/news/2024-03-24/ceo-responds-criticism

Alzheimer's Society. (2024b). *The long goodbye. Our new advert.* https://www.alzheimers.org.uk/about-us/dementia-news-and-media/long-goodbye

Bryden, C. (2005). *Dancing with dementia: My story of living positively with dementia.* London: Jessica Kingsley Publishers.

Bute, J. (2022). *Hello, my name is Jennifer Bute.* Dementia Alliance International. https://dementiaallianceinternational.org/about/resources/our-voice-matters/hello-my-name-is-jennnifer-bute

George, D. R. (2010). The art of medicine overcoming the social death of dementia through language. *The Lancet, 376*(9741), 586–587. https://doi.org/10.1016/S0140-6736(10)61286-X

Horsburgh, T. (2024). *The impact of holding faith, particularly the Christian theologies of hope and suffering, when diagnosed with dementia: An IPA study.* Paisley: University of the West of Scotland.

Johnstone, M.-J. (2016). *Alzheimer's disease, media representations and the politics of euthanasia: Constructing risk and selling death in an ageing society.* Abingdon: Routledge.

Keck, D. (1996). *Forgetting whose we are.* Nashville: Abingdon Press.

Kitwood, T. (1997). *Dementia reconsidered. The person comes first.* Open University Press, Buckingham, Philadelphia.

Low, L., & Purwaningrum, F. (2020). Negative stereotypes, fear and social distance : A systematic review of depictions of dementia in popular culture in the context of stigma. *BMC Geriatrics, 20,* 1–16.

Mitchell, W. (2024). *My final hug in a mug....* Which me am I today? https:// whichmeamitoday.wordpress.com/blog/

Post, S. G. (2002). *The moral challenge of Alzheimer disease: Ethical issues from diagnosis to dying.* Baltimore: JHU Press.

Radden, J., & Fordyce, J. (2006). Into the darkness: Losing identity with dementia. In J. C. Hughes, S. J. Louw, & S. R. Sabat (Eds.), *Dementia: Mind, meaning and the person* (pp. 71–88). Oxford University Press.

Sabat, S. R., & Harrej, R. O. M. (1992). *The construction and deconstruction of self in Alzheimer's disease. Ageing & Society, 12*(4), 443–461.

Simpson, J. (2024). "I still, I still, I still, *I still...* " *The voice of the older person with advanced dementia in residential aged care: An ethnography exploring. What it means for the person to have their Voice* Adelaide: Flinders University. https://theses. flinders.edu.au/view/5c8ad095-c452-4be3-936a-aa2ad1cc8896/1.

Swinton, J. (2017). *Dementia: Living in the memories of God.* SCM Press.

# 4 The cultural struggle in dementia care

## A focus on acculturation, religion and existential concerns

*Önver Cetrez*

### Introduction

In a voluntary work I engage in among Assyrians in Sweden, a Christian minority from the Middle East, we discussed the concerns with dementia care. The participants, all women, demanded more knowledge on dementia. They wanted to know if dementia was affected by the use of medicines. They wanted to understand the symptoms and causes of dementia. They also wanted to know if there was a link to other ill-health conditions. They referred to dementia as "a wicked sickness" (kevo pis) as well as degrading terms used in the community for people with dementia, such as "becoming crazy" (daywanla). Another key concern was the fear of becoming socially isolated and lonely. They expressed their worry of loneliness in a reference to shame. "It is a sin (htitho). She is alone and no one sees after her". They stated that they had not given their parents enough time. Another concern was the fear of becoming passive as one grows older. This was starkly contrasted with an image of having been fully active in their countries of origin, taking care of the household, visiting each other, having a lot of people to interact with. It is notable that emotions related to social relations, existential concerns, and religion were expressed in this short encounter. As the scholarly literature makes clear, cultural and religious attitudes and values, together with misconceptions, stigma and shame, and together with lack of knowledge and lack of information, result in people seeking care only late in the course of dementia (Lang et al., 2017; Low et al., 2011). For migrants and their children, this is complicated by the process of acculturation, in encountering and learning a new culture (Rudmin, 2009), which also has relevance for care-seeking and caregiving. However, the study of dementia care among ethnic minorities with a link to existential concerns needs more attention.

This chapter aims to provide an understanding of the experiences of ethnic minorities in general, without limitation to a specific population, in the context of dementia care. It will examine the experiences of those seeking care, with a particular focus on the influence of culture, acculturation and the concept of existential concerns.

DOI: 10.4324/9781003517733-5

To this end, let us define three key concepts: culture, acculturation and existential. While culture is the way people perceive, interpret and classify the life around them based on their worldview, acculturation refers to a cultural learning process and may come with an experience of stress (Rudmin, 2010). The psychiatrist Irvin D. Yalom has defined humans' existential conflicts in terms of ultimate questions between: life/death, freedom/responsibility, isolation/belonging, and meaning/meaninglessness (1980). The existential has also been associated with activities or expressions of significance, such as rituals (DeMarinis, 2008).

## Stigma and shame in dementia care

Cultural belief systems are a key factor in how we understand a disease, recognize symptoms and decide whether or not to seek care, including for dementia (Khan & Tadros, 2014). The research literature clearly shows several misconceptions about dementia. These include the idea that dementia is primarily part of aging, a mental disorder, a second childhood, a contagious condition, a fate, the work of evil spirits or the evil eye, a lack of faith or a punishment from God (Gove et al., 2016). A substantial body of anthropological and sociological research has identified cultural values, a lack of mastery, productivity, self-control and independence as key factors contributing to the stigma surrounding dementia (Liu et al., 2008). A systematic review of stigma and dementia (Nguyen & Li, 2020) revealed the presence of negative beliefs about people with dementia, stereotypes of dangerousness, loss of self-esteem, lower competence, greater death-thought accessibility and among some non-white populations, as a "white person's illness". The same review revealed the presence of negative emotional reactions, including fear, anxiety, shame, disgust and pity. Additionally, behaviours such as social distance, avoidance, coercion to restrain people with dementia and discrimination were observed. Stigma against people with dementia and their families creates significant barriers to necessary care access and support, ultimately negatively impacting their quality of life. Furthermore, the perceptions and effects of stigma were found to be more intense for ethnic minorities (Nguyen & Li, 2020). The "loss of face" for the afflicted person and family members is experienced as individual shame and guilt, or interpersonally, as a loss of status within a community (Liu et al., 2008).

A study among Chinese and Vietnamese Americans (Liu et al., 2008) showed that dementia-related stigma resembled the stigma of mental illness. This included referring to the afflicted person as crazy, confused, childish or foolish, which resulted in their exclusion from social interactions. The stigma can also extend to the family, as a failure to live up to filial obligations. Despite differences across generations and acculturation levels, Liu et al. assert that one core cultural construct shapes the experience of dementia: the moral status of the family is at stake.

## Presenting late to dementia services

We must tackle the stigma and misconceptions that delay the diagnosis and treatment of dementia. There is a high prevalence of undetected dementia globally, particularly among minority groups (Lang et al., 2017). However, there is a lack of clarity surrounding the causes, which can be attributed to several factors. These include a lack of awareness among GPs (general practitioners) of the symptoms of dementia, insufficient screening and a reluctance to diagnose. Among minorities, a delay in diagnosis is often due to their interpretation of the meaning or severity of dementia symptoms, different methods of help-seeking, poorer ability to negotiate the health system or difficulties among professionals in assessing the cognitive impairment (Low et al., 2011). As previously stated, the misconceptions are that the symptoms of dementia are a normal part of aging or that dementia is linked to a stigmatizing condition, insanity or even a punishment from God. Conversely, studies among Asian Americans demonstrate that perceiving dementia as a normal aspect of aging and avoiding biomedicalization can significantly reduce the stigma attached to dementia, minimize fear and alleviate the burden on caregivers (Liu et al., 2008).

Ethnic differences in the use of dementia services or delays in access to diagnostic services are influenced by several factors, including health literacy, language barriers and differences in healthcare beliefs. Lack of information, poor accessibility to healthcare systems and community expectations of family care obligations also play a role (Czapka & Sagbakken, 2020).

A study on barriers and facilitators in accessing and using dementia care services by minority ethnic groups in Norway (Czapka & Sagbakken, 2020) identified four key themes: a lack of knowledge, a lack of information, cultural factors and barriers related to the healthcare system. The cultural barrier was shaped by religious and other social and moral norms. Examples of cultural barriers included the perception of dementia as a taboo subject, a source of shame for the family, a form of divine punishment, a matter of divine choice or a consequence of one's destiny. Another cultural barrier was related to the family obligation to provide care for the elderly, which is linked to a norm of reciprocity and requires children to care for their elderly parents. Furthermore, the acculturation of younger generations has introduced additional complexity. These individuals have internalized the moral and social norms of both their parents' culture and host culture, creating a dilemma regarding the care of their parents and the question of whether this is primarily the "daughter's" responsibility (p. 9). This can be expressed in terms of a lack of ability to "handle" the situation or a perception that the individual is not up to the task, "she is not good enough", which can lead to feelings of shame (p. 7). In this context, younger generations expressed openness to combining institutional care with family care. One obstacle mentioned in the healthcare system was the possibility of practicing religious rituals.

The study by Mukadam et al. (2011) investigated why ethnic elders present later to dementia services among carers of mixed backgrounds in the UK. The most common reasons were related to forgetfulness; unmanageable symptoms; attribution of symptoms to ageing or physical illness; cultural expectations; expectations that doctors, family members, or religious leaders would guide the caretaker; lack of trust in the healthcare system; other health symptoms or crises precipitating help-seeking and delays in obtaining a diagnosis.

A similar study on barriers to help-seeking highlighted the lack of knowledge and understanding of dementia (Nazir & Kevern, 2024; Kevern et al., 2023). It was not until the dementia was in an advanced stage that outsiders would be approached. An exception was observed among the more acculturated individuals, who demonstrated a diverse and complex understanding. Other reasons included misrecognizing the symptoms of dementia, with a lack of medical labelling of dementia. A poor understanding was also identified as a reason, due to attitudes, assumptions and perceptions of dementia. The decision to seek support first within the family and last from care services presented reasons for the delay. Cultural norms and differences were also identified as barriers, linking to fear of loneliness and losing food preferences and ethnic language.

## Religion's positive and negative effect

Late presentation to dementia services or a reluctance to seek help is also associated with feelings of embarrassment, shame and adherence to religious beliefs. Among Hispanic Americans, there was a tendency to avoid services for cognitively impaired elders due to feelings of embarrassment and a desire to protect the family from shame (Kane, 2000). Furthermore, family secrets were interwoven with religious beliefs, where impairments were attributed to the will of God, to punishment for past sins, to the evil eye or to psychological factors such as nerves. This led to the seeking of coping strategies within these religious domains.

The response of the wider community to dementia, including that of religious leaders, has been observed to be inflexible and lacking in engagement in providing support. This is thought to be due to low levels of awareness and understanding of dementia. This may result in apathy, stigma, and secrecy among those affected (Kevern et al., 2023).

However, the influence of religion on dementia care is not solely negative. A study among Muslim British Pakistanis (Kevern et al., 2023) demonstrated that religious faith provides motivation to care for parents. Furthermore, religious rituals reduced the caregiver burden, releasing anxiety, as expressed by carers: "You find solace in your faith and your religion" (p. 5). Other carers expressed hope of a divine reward.

A study on ethnocultural-sensitive practice and dementia (Kane, 2000) emphasized the importance of recognising the different values, beliefs, behaviours and needs for coping among diverse ethnocultural groups. For instance, a considerable proportion of African-Americans have been observed to rely on informal sources of support and spirituality, with the church representing a particularly visible component of informal support networks. Prayer has been identified as one of the most frequently employed coping strategies among caregivers. In another study, the emotional reactions of lay Arab individuals in Israel to an individual with dementia were measured. The results indicated that higher religiosity was associated with prosocial feelings of compassion and a desire to help, while it was negatively correlated with aggressiveness (Cohen et al., 2009). The authors posited that this is due to the religious belief in Arab society that illness is a matter of God's will or fate and thus outside the realm of personal control, which results in the individual with dementia not being held responsible.

The perception of dementia among general practitioners (white and Asian, in England) was found to manifest as existential anxiety in the context of perceived threat before death. This included fear of dependency, a loss of identity, and a loss of one's personal history and intellect. The latter was expressed as "I wouldn't like to lose myself" (Gove et al., 2016, p. 395). Separating as well as failing to separate between one's existential fear and threat to those of people with dementia, could both contribute towards stigma and need to be recognized.

## Religion as a separate classification

To avoid an overemphasis on a single factor in dementia care, it is recommended that an intersectional approach be adopted, whereby culture, religion, age, gender, education and health literacy are considered as interconnected factors (Czapka & Sagbakken, 2020). Even if an individual knows about dementia but is not able to access services, the issue persists. Alternatively, some individuals may attribute the aetiology of dementia to both neurological and non-neurological factors, such as perceiving dementia as a natural consequence of the ageing process and as a divine will (Khan & Tadros, 2014). Thus, ethnicity as a standalone explanatory factor for the emergence and progression of dementia is problematic. Instead, ethnicity must be considered in conjunction with the process of acculturation.

Similarly, the oversimplification of the relationship between ethnicity, culture, and religion in dementia care among minorities is problematic. Regan (2014) posits that the question of religion should be distinct from culture in general, arguing these should be categorized separately. Earlier research has categorized religiosity as one of numerous culture-related factors. It would be more accurate to classify religion as an equal factor alongside culture, rather than as a sub-factor. One reason for this is that the interpretation of religion varies across different cultures. Furthermore, religion constitutes merely one aspect of an individual's cultural identity. In a review of earlier studies in dementia care among ethnic minorities, Regan identified three specific cultural themes that could be re-classified as religious themes. The first of these was the tendency to understand dementia as God's will and God's plan. This had negative implications for both access to care and care seeking. The second theme was the impact of religious rituals on the behaviour of those with dementia, which led to the conclusion that the house was 'dirty' and therefore in need of cleansing. This, in turn, affected the wider family unit. The third theme was the religious duty or obligation to care for one's family, which was identified as a barrier to accessing external care services until the situation had reached a crisis level (Regan, 2014). As religiously influenced ideologies can impact care-seeking behaviour, Regan suggests that we focus on how religion can contribute to the provision of dementia care services. As an example, scriptures and teachings from various faiths can be a source for stories and sharing of experiences in care-giving. Also, education on the biomedical dimension of dementia can be provided in collaboration with religious leaders to reduce stigma and promote social care services.

## Acculturation relevant to dementia care

Ethnic minority individuals acculturate to their host societies to varying degrees. An understanding of the position of the individual on the acculturation continuum is beneficial to gain insight into their values, norms, communication patterns, behaviours and coping strategies, as these are linked to mental illness and dementia care. Kane (2000) identified culture shock as a factor in the provision of dementia care among Hispanic Americans. Respondents perceived the symptoms to be exacerbated due to feelings of homesickness for cultural food, a lack of access to cultural events, and a lack of exposure to their native language. This is further compounded by younger generations who are either unable or unwilling to assume traditional expectations regarding caregiving, such as the perceived female responsibility. This results in a level of shame and loss of face for the family, with serious implications for the long-term care service continuum. Conversely, among Korean Americans (Jang et al., 2010), being married, having more education, and a higher level of acculturation were found to be associated with increased utilization of dementia-related services.

Knowledge of specific ethnocultural groups is a crucial aspect of effective caregiving. One of the obstacles to effective communication and the accurate diagnosis of symptoms is the presence of cultural differences in the way that symptoms are presented (Khan & Tadros, 2014). This was demonstrated in a Norwegian study on the experiences of health professionals in identifying and diagnosing dementia among immigrants. The study revealed that GPs encountered challenges in assessing dementia among ethnic minority patients, citing language barriers and the lack of culturally appropriate diagnostic tools as significant obstacles (Czapka & Sagbakken, 2020). Furthermore, the acculturation process in the new society, including changes in gender roles and socio-economic status, adds another layer of complexity.

## Conclusions

Notably, there is a paucity of scholarly work on existential concerns and dementia among ethnic minorities. Earlier studies have identified several factors that contribute to the development of anxiety and fear of isolation, loneliness, feelings of insufficiency, shame and guilt. These include a sense of not being able to provide adequate care for one's parents or to conform to the ideals of a strong person. The Assyrian case presented in the introduction provides a further example of these issues. However, on initial examination, this appears to be more a social isolation than an existential one. I. Yalom (1980) would describe existential isolation as a sense of being alone in the world while simultaneously seeking protection, contact and a sense of belonging to a larger entity. Previous research and the brief Assyrian case study have highlighted a significant experience among ethnic minorities: the intricate and demanding nature of acculturation and its connection to stress and dementia. Culture shock, feelings of shame, loosing autonomy, vulnerability, inadequate knowledge and poor language proficiency are significant factors that contribute to the understanding of dementia among ethnic minorities.

In times of crisis, the individual attempts to comprehend and interpret the event. However, for ethnic minorities, the management of crisis occurs concurrently with the process of acculturation. If this process is not effectively managed, it can itself become a source of distress. In such a context, several factors may contribute to the emergence of existential conflicts between isolation and belonging, or freedom and responsibility. These include feelings of guilt, shame, loneliness, fear and a sense of not being able to take responsibility. Previous research has highlighted these factors in different ways. The question for ethnic minorities is not whether these factors contribute to the exacerbation of dementia, but rather how they do so.

## References

Cohen, M., Werner, P., & Azaiza, F. (2009). Emotional reactions of Arab lay persons to a person with Alzheimer's disease. *Aging & Mental Health, 13*(1), 31–37. https://doi.org/10.1080/13607860802154440

Czapka, E. A., & Sagbakken, M. (2020). "It is always me against the Norwegian system." Barriers and facilitators in accessing and using dementia care by minority ethnic groups in Norway: A qualitative study. *BMC Health Services Research, 20*, 954. https://doi.org/10.1186/s12913-020-05801-6.

DeMarinis, V. (2008). The impact of postmodernization on existential health in Sweden: Psychology of religion's function in existential public health analysis. *Archive for the Psychology of Religion, 30*, 57–74.

Gove, D., Downs, M., Vernooij-Dassen, M., & Small, N. (2016). Stigma and GPs' perceptions of dementia. *Aging & Mental Health, 20*(4), 391–400. https://doi.org/10.1080/13607863.2015.1015962.

Jang, Y., Kim, G., & Chiriboga, D. (2010). Knowledge of Alzheimer's disease, feelings of shame, and awareness of services among Korean American elders. *Journal of Aging and Health, 22*(4), 419–433. https://doi.org/10.1177/0898264309360672.

Kane, M. N. (March/April 2000). Ethnoculturally-sensitive practice and Alzheimer's disease. *American Journal of Alzheimer's Disease*, 80–86.

Kevern, P., Lawrence, D., Nazir, N., & Tsaroucha, A. (2023). Religious influences on the experience of family carers of people with dementia in a British Pakistani Muslim community. *Healthcare, 11*, 120. https://doi.org/10.3390/healthcare11010120.

Khan, F., & Tadros, G. (2014). Complexity in cognitive assessment of elderly British minority ethnic groups: Cultural perspective. *Dementia, 13*(4), 467–482. https://doi.org/10.1177/1471301213475539.

Lang, L., Clifford, A., Wei, L., et al. (2017). Prevalence and determinants of undetected dementia in the community: A systematic literature review and a meta-analysis. *BMJ Open 7*, e011146. https://doi.org/10.1136/bmjopen-2016-011146.

Liu, D., Hinton, L., Tran, C., Hinton, D., & Barker, J. C. (2008). Reexamining the relationships among dementia, stigma, and aging in immigrant Chinese and Vietnamese family caregivers. *Journal of Cross-Cultural Gerontology, 23*(3), 283–299. https://doi.org/10.1007/s10823-008-9075-5.

Low, L. F., Anstey, K. J., Lackersteen, S. M. P., & Camit, M. (2011). Help-seeking and service use for dementia in Italian, Greek and Chinese Australians. *Aging & Mental Health, 15*(3), 397–404. https://doi.org/10.1080/13607863.2010.536134.

Mukadam, N., Cooper, C., Basit, B., & Livingston, G. (2011). Why do ethnic elders present later to UK dementia services? A qualitative study. *International Psychogeriatrics, 23*(7), 1070–1077. https://doi.org/10.1017/S1041610211000214.

Nazir, N., & Kevern, P. (2024). Understanding and awareness of dementia in the Pakistani-origin community of stoke-on-trent, UK: A scenario-based interview study. *Healthcare, 12*(2), 251. https://doi.org/10.3390/healthcare12020251.

Nguyen, T., & Li, X. (2020). Understanding public-stigma and self-stigma in the context of dementia: A systematic review of the global literature. *Dementia, 19*(2), 148–181. https://doi.org/10.1177/1471301218800122.

Regan, J. L. (2014). Redefining dementia care barriers for ethnic minorities: The religion–culture distinction. *Mental Health, Religion & Culture, 17*(4), 345–353. https://doi.org/10.1080/13674676.2013.805404.

Rudmin, F. W. (2010). Phenomenology of acculturation: Retrospective reports from the Philippines, Japan, Quebec, and Norway. *Culture & Psychology, 16*(3), 313–332. https://doi.org/10.1177/1354067X10371139.

Rudmin, F. (2009). Constructs, measurements and models of acculturation and acculturative stress. *International Journal of Intercultural Relations, 33*, 106–123.

Yalom, I. D. (1980). *Existential psychotherapy.* New York: Basic Books.

# 5 Vignettes

## Existential dramas in patients with severe dementia

*Tor-Arne Isene*

For people with severe dementia, time consists of fleeting moments. What happens here and now may be forgotten and lost from memory shortly afterward. However, those who care for people with dementia can view these fleeting moments as more than just transient experiences. They are small pieces in a larger picture, revolving around what is important to these individuals – what it is that may give meaning to life. This chapter is based on a study about 'Meaning in life for people with severe dementia' (Isene et al., 2021, 2022). In one of the published articles from this study, we encounter 'Anne', 'Gerda', 'Emma' and 'David', whom I have chosen to call them, and who are patients with severe dementia in a dementia ward. These encounters are narratives from their everyday situations that can illustrate for us what existential meaning in life for people with severe dementia can be about.

As a participant observer, I had the opportunity to follow patients with severe dementia over extended periods of time. The staff at the dementia ward did an admirable job focusing on well-being, security and individual presence. Part of their approach involved initiating meaningful activities where patients engaged in daily chores, such as folding laundry, setting the table before meals, or helping with gardening. In my observational role, I had plenty of time to follow the individual patients even during seemingly uneventful periods or when no specific interventions occurred. Surprisingly, these seemingly idle moments were not empty; they held their own unique content. Much of what I observed was about short, often fleeting moments. Some anxiety, longing, loss and confusion – but also 'golden moments' with experiences of calm, well-being, connection and contentment. I witnessed how people with severe dementia could experience everyday life, that it could be understood as being about experiencing meaning in life.

Communicating about existential topics with people with dementia can be a very difficult task. One of the reasons for this, I believe, is that when we talk about the existential, we tend to relate to it in a very cognitive and abstract way, which is problematic when cognitive capacity is deficient. However,

DOI: 10.4324/9781003517733-6

experiencing meaning in life is vital for all people, which means that people with dementia also need to understand the world around them. This is what is at stake in the narratives presented here, the experience of existential meaning, which is why the narratives are termed *existential dramas*.[1]

## Anne

In an encounter with Anne, we gain insight into how, for a brief moment, she experiences a deep existential pain over the fact that the people who have been close to her are gone, and she feels old and alone. What triggered this realization in Anne was a joyful event where her birthday was celebrated. Anne usually had a cheerful mind and believed that she was young and that her parents were still alive. However, this morning was different.

I am sitting with Anne in her room. She is complaining a little about her aching legs and back, after the morning care. Then one of the carers enters the room approaching Anne. 'Today is the fifteenth of October! Do you know whose birthday it is today?' the carer asks. Anne, who until now has been sitting slumped and sleepily in her chair, lightens up. 'The fifteenth of October...' she says smiling. 'It is your birthday today, Anne!' the carer continues. 'Yes, it is,' Anne replies. A second carer enters the room and the three of us are standing in front of Anne dancing and singing a birthday song. Anne covers her mouth and nose with both hands. She is smiling, and tears appear in her eyes. 'Thank you so much' she says emphasizing each word. One of the carers leaves the room and comes back with a tiny flag she puts on the table.

The carers have left. Anne and I are sitting alone in her room. She is holding a cup of hot chocolate and sits thoughtfully in silence. Tears start flowing from her eyes. I move closer to her and put my hand on her back. 'You look sad' I say to her, 'Are you thinking of something?'. 'Yes. Home.' She looks at me, 'I am thinking of those back home. They are gone. I am old.' 'Yes, you are eighty-three years old today. That is a high age,' I say to her. 'Yes,' she replies. 'It is.'

Then Anne becomes quiet again. She is complaining a little bit about her aching back again and expresses that her pains are strong today.

## Gerda

Losing her grip on her identity was a constant struggle for Gerda. She often sought solitude and exclaimed 'I can't do anything anymore'. Experiencing functional impairment and loss in coping and cognitive capacity, her use of 'anymore' indicates that she was grieving the person she used to be. However, it seems that her body was able to help her connect to her background and make a transformation from a crisis of meaning into an experience of meaningfulness.

Gerda had been very anxious in the morning. Three times during breakfast she had left the dining room and gone back to her room. After breakfast, baking traditional Christmas cookies was on the agenda. The dining room was cleared and prepared for baking cookies. Cookie dough was already prepared in a bowl on the table. Gerda was invited to join the baking activity. She first excused herself saying 'I don't know how to bake cookies anymore.' But eventually, she came along.

Carefully entering the dining room, Gerda noticed the cookie dough on the table. She went to the table, picked up a knife and started to cut the cookie dough into smaller pieces. I put an apron over her head, and she tied it, without looking, with a knot on her back within seconds. The anxious insecure woman was now in charge and in command of baking Christmas cookies. Together with one of the other patients, they rolled, sliced, put the cookies on a baking tray, brushed them with eggs and sprinkled them with chopped almonds. Within 15 minutes several trays of cookies were ready for the oven. The temperature in the oven was set to 200 degrees Celsius, and when Gerda stood in front of the oven, she commented that it was set too high and should be lowered to 180 degrees.

## Emma

Emma had trouble speaking but could express herself in short sentences of two or three words at a time. She often couldn't recall the words she wanted to use. Several years ago, Emma had sung in a choir for many years. This experience with choir practice from earlier in her life turned out to give Emma an unexpected opportunity of being able to communicate.

One afternoon in December Emma went together with one other dementia patient and two carers to a cafeteria. This was on the St. Lucia day and an invited choir performed a Lucia celebration in the cafeteria. As we sat drinking coffee at a table, the doors opened, and the choir entered the room in a procession wearing white robes and holding candles in their hands. They were singing the St. Lucia hymn as they entered the room.

As the choir entered the cafeteria, Emma stood up from her chair and almost in a spellbound manner watched and listened to the choir in the procession. Emma started to hum along with the choir.

After finishing the procession, the choir held a little concert in the cafeteria, singing a few Christmas carols. Emma was standing a few meters in front of the choir. She was humming along with the choir and slowly moved the body to the music. After a few songs Emma started to hum the alto voice to one of the carols.

Emma's experiences of choir rehearsals and meeting the Lucia Choir suggest that music and singing are an important source of meaning for her. Another source of meaning for Emma is her connection to nature and the joy of staying physically fit outdoors. One morning, when Emma was not feeling well and was struggling with anxiety and despair, it turned out that her connection to nature was making a difference for her.

> Emma was sitting in a chair in the living room. She was crying, and a carer was sitting next to her, trying to comfort her. I sat down with them. 'Life is over now' Emma said. For a moment she was sitting in silence with us. Then suddenly she got up, left the living room and started wandering down the corridor. 'It will pass when I am allowed to be alone by myself!' she said.
>
> After walking up and down the corridor for a few minutes, Emma came over to me, looked into my eyes and asked, 'isn't there anything to do when things are like this?'. I asked her back 'is there something you like to do, when things are like this?'. 'I like going for long walks,' she answered. 'Good! Then the two of us can go outside for a walk' I answered.
>
> We put on outdoor clothing and went outside. The rain was pouring down. We stood outside the front door and I asked her if she wanted to wait until the rain had stopped. 'It doesn't matter!' she replied and started walking out in the rain.
>
> It was late in the autumn and we walked carefully on the icy and slippery roads. Most of the time we were walking in silence without talking. 'Awful weather!' Emma exclaimed a couple of times. At the same time, it appeared that her mood was lightening as we were walking in the rain. After fifteen minutes' walk in the rain, we returned to the ward. We were cold and soaking wet to the skin. 'Was it okay to walk in the rain?' I asked her when we came inside. 'It was wonderful,' she answered with a smile and appeared to be very pleased.

## David

Over the last few months, David's dementia had become much worse, leading to a substantial decline in his ability to function. He kept saying 'Sorry' or 'I'm sorry', which was often perceived by those around him as a kind of tic because of its constant nature. However, given the significant functional decline David had recently experienced, which had led to major changes in the daily lives of his wife and himself, could his repeated apologies be an expression of an existential crisis? Engaging him in familiar and meaningful activities seemed to make a positive difference.

> One afternoon David was sitting in his room, drinking a cup of coffee. The gardener had just mowed the lawn outside, and I suggested to David

that we could go outside to collect the grass from the lawn. At first, he declined, but then he decided to come along as one of the carers and I went outside into the garden. He said 'sorry' several times on our way outside. The lawn was divided into sections between the walking paths. David fetched a rake and started raking the grass together with habitual movements. I was working close by. David was thorough and systematic. Every time we moved to a new section; he started raking by himself without further instructions. After raking the grass into small piles, he asked for something to put the grass in. One of the other patients was operating the wheelbarrow, and the two of them were cooperating smoothly. 'It is fun to rake!' David said and appeared to be very pleased. There were no 'sorry's at all when we were outside in the garden working together.

## Meaning embodied

The stories give us small glimpses of how people with severe dementia can experience and deal with existential meaning in everyday life. These small glimpses are important because immediate experiences are connected to something meaningful from the past, something larger and more fundamental. Linking experiences and events across time integrating the past with the present, provides experiences of meaning (Baumeister et al., 2013, p. 509). Living with dementia makes abstract thinking less accessible (American Psychiatric Association [APA], 2013; World Health Organization [WHO], 2017), making it difficult to consciously search for meaning. But in the situations described in this chapter, we see that the body is able to take on this role. In Gerda's story, it is the body's procedural memory that remembers how to bake Christmas cookies, helping her to connect with the strong traditions associated with Christmas preparations, which are seen as an important source of meaning (Schnell, 2009, 2021). In Emma's stories, we again see her using her body to communicate with the Lucia choir, using her senses and responding to the music. It is by connecting to nature, exposing her body to the rain on that harsh autumn day, that she manages to get out of her anxiety and despair. David experiences a sense of coping that contrasts sharply with his loss of function. And for Anne, we may wonder whether it is the pain in her back or the existential pain of feeling old and abandoned that is stronger.

Meaning-making for people with dementia is not a cognitive exercise but takes place in interactions with others. The people in these stories experienced the situations through their bodies, and it is highly unlikely that they would have even considered that what they were experiencing was about meaning in life. However, for the people around them, who relate to them and care for them, it is helpful to understand and interpret these events existentially as being about meaning in life. The existential dramas address coherence, significance, orientation and belonging, which are the key concepts for experiencing meaning in life (Schnell, 2009, 2021; Schnell & Danbolt, 2023).

A shift in focus from the purely verbal to the practical and concrete, such as the existential dramas outlined in this chapter, can help us to connect with the existential themes experienced by people with dementia. Acknowledging the embodied nature of individuals provides a lens through which to explore the expressions of meaning in life that can be observed within the hidden realities of dementia. Recognizing people with dementia as whole human beings, with a profound awareness of their existential dimension, enhances the dignity and importance of person-centred dementia care. This perspective underscores the necessity of prioritizing health policy aspects, such as funding and resource allocation, to support this essential practice.

Caring for someone with dementia involves experiences of falling short, of having to endure chaos and meaninglessness between meaningful moments. However, I hope that the existential dramas in this chapter will encourage us to seek out and identify experiences of meaning in the lives of those we care for. Despite cognitive shortcomings, the body retains the ability to bridge the past with the present, providing experiences of being useful, contributing, demonstrating skill, and so on. This opens up the possibility of what meaning in life a person with severe dementia can maintain and experience. By respecting, following, and being close and present, we can better understand where the person with dementia is at the moment. The etymological meaning of *respect* (re- "back" + specere "to look at") means to see again, to see once more. This encourages us to look beyond the symptoms of dementia and seek to find the existential meaning in how a person with severe dementia experiences and understands the world.

## Note

1 The narratives presented in this chapter were first published in Isene, T.-A., Thygesen, H., Danbolt, L. J., & Stifoss-Hanssen, H. (2022). Embodied meaning-making in the experiences and behaviours of persons with dementia [Original research]. *Dementia, 21* (2), 442–456. https://doi.org/10.1177/14713012211042979

## References

American Psychiatric Association (APA) (2013). *Diagnostic and statistical manual of mental disorders: DSM-5* (5th ed.). Washington DC: American Psychiatric Association.
Baumeister, R. F., Vohs, K. D., Aaker, J. L., & Garbinsky, E. N. (2013). Some key differences between a happy life and a meaningful life. *The Journal of Positive Psychology, 8*(6), 505–516. https://doi.org/10.1080/17439760.2013.830764
Isene, T.-A., Kjørven Haug, S. H., Stifoss-Hanssen, H., Danbolt, L. J., Ødbehr, L. S., & Thygesen, H. (2021). Meaning in life for patients with severe dementia: A qualitative study of healthcare professionals' Interpretations [Original Research]. *Frontiers in Psychology, 12*(3734). https://doi.org/10.3389/fpsyg.2021.701353
Isene, T.-A., Thygesen, H., Danbolt, L. J., & Stifoss-Hanssen, H. (2022). Embodied meaning-making in the experiences and behaviours of persons with dementia [Original research]. *Dementia, 21*(2), 442–456. https://doi.org/10.1177/14713012211042979

Schnell, T. (2009). The sources of meaning and meaning in life questionnaire (SoMe): Relations to demographics and well-being. *The Journal of Positive Psychology, 4*(6), 483–499. https://doi.org/10.1080/17439760903271074

Schnell, T. (2021). *The psychology of meaning in life* (T. Schnell, Trans.; 1st ed.). London/New York: Routledge.

Schnell, T., & Danbolt, L. J. (2023). The Meaning and Purpose Scales (MAPS): Development and multi-study validation of short measures of meaningfulness, crisis of meaning, and sources of purpose. *BMC Psychology, 11*(1), 304. https://doi.org/10.1186/s40359-023-01319-8

World Health Organization (WHO) (2017). *Global action plan on the public health response to dementia 2017–2025*. Geneva: World Health Organization.

**Part II**

**Existential health related to person-centered care, brain complexity of dementia, daily living and emotions**

# 6  Person-centred care and existential health

*Bjørn Lichtwarck*

## Introduction

Tom Kitwood stated in 1997 in his seminal work, Dementia Reconsidered, that

> there is, however, a very sombre point to consider about contemporary practice. It is that a man or a woman could be given the most accurate diagnosis, subjected to the most thorough assessment, provided with a highly detailed care plan, and given a place in the most pleasant surroundings – without any meeting of the I-Thou kind ever having taken place.
>
> (Kitwood, 1997)

By this statement, Kitwood coins the two very essential ideas of what person-centred care (PCC) is about: to see the person first, despite any functional or cognitive impairments, and second, to emphasise the person's existential experience in a relational frame with others. The "I-Thou" meeting stands in contrast to the "I-It" meeting, where the person with dementia is reduced to the "It", e.g., to be a patient, a resident, a dement, a sufferer, an Alzheimer victim, etc. In this chapter, I will therefore develop further on Tom Kitwood's and Steven Sabat's existential concept of being a person and of personhood, which is so central to understand PCC (Kitwood, 1997; Sabat, 2006). I will show how these concepts are associated with the three main dimensions of existential health: meaningfulness, crises of meaning, and sources of meaning. Finally, I will discuss in which way these concepts from existential health can enrich person-centred care in practice and discuss which factors promote or hinder the integration of PCC and existential health care into standard care practices. But first, is there a uniform definition or conception of person-centred care?

## What is person-centred care?

Even though PCC can be considered as one of the most influential care practice philosophies or frameworks for a value-based dementia care practice, there is

DOI: 10.4324/9781003517733-8

no universally used definition or common understanding of the concept PCC. Since the 1990s, the social-psychologist Tom Kitwood started to use the term person-centred care in relation to care for people with dementia and published a series of papers constructing both the philosophical concept PCC and the care framework of PCC (Kitwood, 1990, 1995). Central in his work was the theoretical concept of personhood. Personhood was defined by Kitwood as the "standing or status that is bestowed upon one human being, by others, in the context of relationship and social being" (Kitwood, 1997). And he added: "it implies recognition, respect and trust". To develop this definition, he drew on transcendental discourses asserting that "being-in-itself is sacred", ethical discourses proclaiming that "each person has absolute value", and social psychology perspectives linking a person's self-esteem to assigned roles and their place within the social context (Kitwood, 1997). As such, PCC is, according to Kitwood, most of all a concept involving the person's relations with others, and not to be confused with individual care or patient-centred care, the two latter concepts being just a part of person-centred care. Sabat used the Zulu proverb: "Umuntu ngumuntu ngabantu" meaning "a person is a person through others" to explain to what extent the character of our meetings with the person with dementia could have a profoundly negative or positive effect on the person with dementia (Sabat, 2006). The character of these meetings could impact on the person's subjective experience of having dementia, on the person's possibility to still display his remaining cognitive abilities, to meet the demands of everyday life and finally the person's quality of life and his or her possibility to discover meaning in life (Sabat, 2006). The challenge, but also the opportunity, is that these meetings happen several times a day, every day in nursing homes, especially in the care interactions between the staff and the residents.

However, the translation of theoretical concepts into practice is easier said than done. To clarify and to make the concept of PCC more comprehensible and practically implementable, Brooker and Latam developed the VIPS framework (Brooker & Latham, 2016). VIPS is an acronym for; V: Valuing the person with dementia independent of the person's functional or cognitive level; I: an Individual approach based on the person's resources, values, and preferences; P: always try to take the person's Perspective and try to interpret this perspective, and S: to develop a supportive Social environment preserving old relationships and creating new ones, to fulfil the person's psychological and social needs. For each of these four dimensions six so-called indicators are developed, to be used in daily practice to evaluate and develop PCC in the nursing homes (Brooker & Latham, 2016). To further ease the translation of the VIPS framework into practice, several practice models or care programs have been developed, e.g., VIPS practice model and the TIME model (Targeted interdisciplinary model for Evaluation and Treatment of neuropsychiatric symptoms) (Lichtwarck et al., 2018; Rokstad et al., 2013). However, one of the main challenges in nursing homes is the complex social, psychological, and physical situation for the residents. How does PCC embrace these complex needs?

## Person-centred care and the need for a bio-psychosocial approach

People with dementia who live in nursing homes are usually over 80 years old and have several chronic medical conditions, so-called multimorbidity. They also frequently display diverse behavioural and psychological symptoms (BPSD) (Helvik, Selbæk, Saltyte Benth, Røen, & Bergh, 2018). BPSD is a common term for a wide range of symptoms like agitation, aggression, symptoms of psychosis, affective symptoms (anxiety and depression), and apathy. Most nursing home residents die in nursing homes, and the most common underlying cause of death is dementia (Vossius, Bergh, Selbæk, Lichtwarck, & Myhre, 2022). In addition, since the dementia syndrome represents different brain diseases which nearly all are progressive and lead towards a state of complete dependence for the patients of the staff in the nursing homes, this places high demands on both the competence of the staff and adequate staffing in nursing homes. This portray of the complex health and care situation for the nursing home resident represents the "ugliness" of the dementia syndrome and will naturally for most residents have a major bearing on the content of person-centred care and on which existential questions that emerge as important for the residents. When pain dominates the daily life for a resident, pain relief, the meaning of pain, and consolation become the overarching thoughts and needs for the patient. When feeling alone and isolated, because of difficulties or obstacles to going outside the nursing home, the need for assistance, comfort, interest, and love from the staff become imperative. Person-centred care models, frameworks, or programs which do not take into consideration a broad comprehensive approach including both biological, psychological, and social factors will usually fall short. In the next paragraphs, I will discuss how existential concepts can and should be entrenched in this bio-psychosocial PCC approach.

## How can dimensions of the existential concept of meaning in life enrich and complement person-centred care?

Meaningfulness, crisis of meaning and sources of meaning constitute the three main dimensions of the existential concept of meaning in life according to Schnell (Schnell, 2020). She describes meaningfulness as the "basic trust that life is worth living", stemming from our often unconscious perception of life as coherent, significant, oriented and accompanied by a sense of belonging (Schnell, 2009). The description of meaningfulness is conveyed without the condition of having a cognitive awareness for the person itself on what it is that creates or are the sources of meaning. This is of importance for people with dementia living in nursing homes, since many of them have severe cognitive impairments (Isene et al., 2021). It implies that the role of the staff in contributing to meaningfulness for these residents is even more important than for residents without dementia. PCC when applied and integrated in practice can be a powerful tool towards meaningfulness. As I will discuss later in this chapter, the staff needs an awareness on the importance and power that lies in their hands to contribute to meaning in life for the residents. I will describe how being aware of the dimensions of meaningfulness could enrich and widening their repertoire when practicing PCC (Isene et al., 2021).

*Coherence* in life is strongly attributed to the person's sense of identity, sensing that even if we develop and change through the years, there is a continuity with the past for whom we are as a person. The "I" in the VIPS framework emphasises the importance of Individual care based on the person's values, preferences, and remaining resources. To develop this dimension of PCC there is a need for the staff to gain knowledge of the person's biography including these aspects (Brooker & Latham, 2016). Coherence for the person with dementia also means that daily activities in the person's daily life reflect who the person is and the person's identity, supporting coherence in the present (Kitwood, 1997). This can, for example, be done by creating individualised care plans, an essential part of the "I" in the VIPS framework.

Valuing people with dementia, the "V" in VIPS, has a broader meaning beyond the individual, but, of course, also has an important impact on the individual person in nursing homes. Valuing the person with dementia is an important contribution to the sense of being a *significant* person for others and being seen and treated like someone significant regardless of the person's cognitive or functional abilities. This should imply that the person with dementia has the same rights as everybody else to fulfil their lives, to be treated with respect, and to make choices and decisions in life, to not be subjected to unnecessary coercion, being locked in, not being able to get out when needed, etc. (De Sabbata, 2020). In this way, the "V" in the VIPS framework and the concept "significant" in meaningfulness have consequences for both the organisation and resource availability for people with dementia living in nursing homes.

Can life be *oriented* for the person with dementia, as a concept of meaningfulness? And how does this concept relate to the VIPS framework? This seems difficult to imagine if "oriented" is defined as having precise long-term goals and objectives. But if "oriented" relates to the sense of coherence with the past and the acceptance and the adaption to the present situation, life can be "oriented". In a recent interview study of ten residents with mild to severe dementia, the participants intertwined the past and present and expressed an acceptance of their present situation with the help of the past (Nylund et al., 2025).

Again, the person's life history becomes essential and can be used in the interactions with the residents as an instrument for the staff to contribute to both identity and orientation in life.

The social perspective in the VIPS framework relates particularly to the concept of *belonging* in meaningfulness. The definition of personhood by Kitwood emphasises this social aspect of being a person. The meetings with the person with dementia, as discussed initially in this chapter, should be of the character "I-Though meeting", not a superficial, brief, and impersonal "I-It meeting". For those residents who still have family and close relationships, these meetings are often mentioned as one of the most important sources of meaningfulness (Nylund et al., 2025). This underscores the social aspects of the VIPS framework. For many residents with dementia belonging is also strongly connected to their relationship with staff. To enhance a sense of belonging for the residents this implies taking a step away from "the us and them" mentality. This means in practice, for example, sharing meals together, participating together in common meaningful activities like preparing meals, cleaning and changing the bedding, dusting in the nursing home unit, mopping the floor, etc. (Kitwood, 1995). Evidently, some of these activities are not possible for some people with severe dementia, but to my experience, even if they cannot fully participate, they can be part of the activity talking to and watching the staff and those who can participate. To make this happen the nursing home units must be adequately staffed, since sharing activities take time and cannot be done under time pressure with the risk of outpacing the residents.

## Crisis of meaning, positioning, and malignant social psychology

The second dimension, crisis of meaning, refers to the perception of one's life as empty and devoid of meaning (Schnell, 2020). This can happen when your expectations and needs are not adequately met or when few of the sources of meaning are present (see paragraph below). In PCC, the notion "malignant social psychology" refers to negative attitudes and actions from the staff towards the residents and could easily lead to a crisis of meaning (Kitwood, 1997). These attitudes and actions could have a detrimental effect on person's personhood. Kitwood lists a range of such behaviours like treachery and deception, disempowerment, infantilisation, intimidation, labelling, outpacing, banishment, objectification, ignoring, mockery, etc. He emphasised that this often is due to a cultural heritage, and not as intendant evil actions from the staff. This cultural heritage is most often present where the care culture is influenced by fear, anonymity, and an extreme power imbalance in favour of the staff (Kitwood, 1997). Sabat used the term "positioning" of the person in this regard, meaning that nearly all actions or reactions from the person with dementia are attributed to their dementia disease (Sabat, 2006). When a person with dementia shows anger or agitation, does not cooperate with the staff or their next of kin, or always wants things done in their own ways, these actions are then interpreted as symptoms of the brain disease and not legitimate actions or reactions from the person with dementia. Low levels of skills and competence, along with understaffing, increase the risk of malignant social psychology and the development of crises of meaning among the residents.

It should nevertheless be noted that a crisis of meaning and changes in behaviour and psychological symptoms can be the result of the dementia itself, the brain disease with its neurological changes affecting the person resulting in cognitive decline, the loss of daily living functions, and finally not being able to live at home as before. Even the very best and adopted person-centred care from the caregivers and all available sources of meaning cannot always prevent a crisis. But comfort and support can always be given. This emphasises that crises of meaning have multiple causes, though they usually are a result of the interactions between the person's neurological and cognitive changes and how the person is met by their environment (Kitwood, 1997).

## Sources of meaning and person-centred activities

Sources of meaning encompass experiences or activities that provide life with meaning. This should be activities based on the person's remaining resources, interests, and preferences and customised to the person (Kitwood, 1997). This can include activities ranging from comfort and wellness activities, participation in daily tasks, physical exercises, be read for sessions, walks, and taking part in rituals such as church services, birthdays, etc. Care practice models such as the TIME model and the VIPS practice model, which both are based on the VIPS framework, can help the staff arrive at a common and shared understanding of the person's situation, and agree upon which activities that are most suitable to suggest for the individual resident (Lichtwarck et al., 2018; Rokstad et al., 2013).

The activity "The I and Though meeting", i.e., the meeting between the staff and the residents during everyday life interactions, as described earlier, can however be the most important source of meaning for the residents. Spontaneous conversations, during care situations, when the caregiver knows the patient's life history and is aware of the importance of the moments in this conversation, can have an impact on all the dimensions of meaning in life. A qualitative study based on interviews with 31 nurses from four Norwegian nursing homes used the term "being present" and "sensitivity in communication" to characterise conversations with the residents that could strengthen the residents' personhood and incorporate spiritual care (Ødbehr, Kvigne, Hauge, & Danbolt, 2015). In a qualitative explorative study on how the staff interpret the residents' experience of meaning in life, this awareness was described as "being on a treasure hunt" for what is important for the resident, and "catching the moment" in these everyday situations. (Isene et al., 2021). The authors added that being able to develop the staff's skills and awareness of these possibilities in the daily caring for the residents, there is a need for increased resources and competence building in nursing homes.

## Conclusion and implications for practice

In this chapter, I have demonstrated that there is considerable correspondence between the concepts of the VIPS framework in PCC and the dimensions of existential health and meaning in life as described by Schnell (Schnell, 2020). In addition, I have argued that an increased awareness by the staff of the existential dimensions meaningfulness, crises of meaning, and sources of meaning can enrich PCC, and can provide the staff with a better justification of the various concepts in PCC. The main challenge however is the translation of this knowledge into daily practice in the care for people with dementia. Several care practice models have been developed to ease the translation of the concept of PCC to the everyday care practice (Lichtwarck et al., 2018; Rokstad et al., 2013). We need a boost both at the societal level and within individual organisations and workplaces to enhance the quality of care for people with dementia, and to implement PCC more effectively in practice, for example, through these care practice models. We have the knowledge, it's time to implement it.

## References

Brooker, D., & Latham, I. (2016). *Person-centred dementia care: Making services better with the VIPS framework (2.utg.)* (2 ed.). London: Jessica Kingsley Publishers.
De Sabbata, K. (2020). Dementia, treatment decisions, and the UN convention on the rights of persons with disabilities. A new framework for old problems. *Frontiers in Psychiatry, 11*, 571722. doi:10.3389/fpsyt.2020.571722
Helvik, A., Selbæk, G., Saltyte Benth, J., Røen, I., & Bergh, S. (2018). *The course of neuropsychiatric symptoms in nursing home residents from admission to 30-month follow-up. PLoS One, 13*(10), e0206147. doi:10.1371/journal.pone.0206147.
Isene, T.-A., Kjørven Haug, S. H., Stifoss-Hanssen, H., Danbolt, L. J., Ødbehr, L. S., & Thygesen, H. (2021). Meaning in life for patients with severe dementia: A qualitative study of healthcare professionals' interpretations. *Frontiers in Psychology, 12*. doi:10.3389/fpsyg.2021.701353
Kitwood, T. (1990). The dialectics of dementia: With particular reference to Alzheimer's disease. *Ageing & Society, 10*(2), 177–196.
Kitwood, T. (1995). Cultures of care: Tradition and change. In T. Kitwood & S. Benson (Eds.), *The new culture of dementia care* (pp. 8–11). London: Hawker Publications.
Kitwood, T. (1997). *Dementia reconsidered – The person comes first.* Birmingham: Open University Press.

Lichtwarck, B., Selbaek, G., Kirkevold, O., Rokstad, A. M. M., Benth, J. S., Lindstrom, J. C., & Bergh, S. (2018). Targeted interdisciplinary model for evaluation and treatment of neuropsychiatric symptoms: A cluster randomized controlled trial. *American Journal of Geriatric Psychiatry, 26*(1), 25–38. doi:10.1016/j.jagp.2017.05.015

Nylund, S., Danbolt, L. J., Feiring, I. H., Bergh, S., Lichtwarck, B., Kirkevold, Ø., & Hestad, K. (2025). Meaning in life for residents with dementia living in long-term nursing homes: An exploratory qualitative interview-based study (Under Review). *Archives for the Psychology of Religion.*

Ødbehr, L. S., Kvigne, K., Hauge, S., & Danbolt, L. J. (2015). Spiritual care to persons with dementia in nursing homes; a qualitative study of nurses and care workers experiences. *BMC Nursing, 14*, 70. doi:10.1186/s12912-015-0122-6

Rokstad, A. M., Rosvik, J., Kirkevold, O., Selbaek, G., Saltyte Benth, J., & Engedal, K. (2013). The effect of person-centred dementia care to prevent agitation and other neuropsychiatric symptoms and enhance quality of life in nursing home patients: A 10-month randomized controlled trial. *Dementia & Geriatric Cognitive Disorders, 36*(5–6), 340–353. doi:10.1159/000354366

Sabat, S. R. (2006). Mind, meaning and personhood in dementia: The effects of positioning. In J. C. Hughes, S. J. Louw, & S. R. Sabat (Eds.), *Dementia: Mind, meaning, and the person* (pp. 287–302). Oxford: Ocford University Press.

Schnell, T. (2009). The Sources of Meaning and Meaning in Life Questionnaire (SoMe): Relations to demographics and well-being. *The Journal of Positive Psychology, 4*(6), 483–499.

Schnell, T. (2020). *The psychology of meaning in life* (1 ed.). New York: Routledge.

Vossius, C., Bergh, S., Selbæk, G., Lichtwarck, B., & Myhre, J. (2022). Cause and place of death in Norwegian nursing home residents. *Scandinavian Journal of Public Health,* 14034948221140195. doi:10.1177/14034948221140195

# 7 The brain and the complexity of dementia

*Sverre Bergh*

## The brain

The brain is a small organ in the human body, roughly the size of two clenched fists. Nevertheless, it is one of the most complex organs in the human body. The more than 100 billion neurones are interconnected in synapses. Each neurone has 1,000–15,000 synapses. So, there are an almost unbelievable high number of connections in the brain. This complexity in the brain is needed to perform all the complex tasks in the body, like muscle movement; breathing; elimination; producing, regulating, and distributing hormones; cognitive functions; affections; and personality. Different brain diseases will affect the function of the body in different ways, e.g., a stroke can impair skin sensation, muscle movement, and the ability to speech.

Cognition covers functions as memory, attention, executive function, and language. Cognitive impairment may be caused by factors such as neurodegeneration and aging, vascular diseases, hypoxia to the brain, traumatic brain injury, depression, and medical treatment. Any damage to the brain will change the function of the brain, depending on the location and size of the damage. Damaged neurons cannot regenerate. But the damaged areas can reorganize, and other parts of the brain can replace the functions of the damaged areas. This phenomenon is called plasticity and can be seen after traumatic brain injuries and strokes. Rehabilitation is therefore important and should be offered to persons with brain diseases.

## What is dementia?

The European population is ageing. Projections indicate that the share of people over 65 years could reach 30% of the EU population by 2030, as opposed to 10% in 1960 (Kiss, 2020). With an increasing number of older people, symptoms, syndromes, and disease following old age will increase in numbers and severity. Cognitive impairment and dementia are among the most prevalent diseases in the older population. The dementia syndrome is hallmarked by decreased memory, loss of initiative, decreased cognitive- and

DOI: 10.4324/9781003517733-9

motor speed, reduced problem-solving capacity, and language problems (Gale et al., 2018). All these symptoms can be associated with reduced capacity to take part in social, physical, and entertaining activities. With decreased memory, loss of language, and a shift from abstract to concrete thinking, defining and describing the meaning in life may be difficult as the dementia progresses.

Dementia can be caused by a range of diseases, where Alzheimer's disease is the most common. Other pathologies that can cause dementia are vascular dementia, Lewy body dementias, and frontotemporal dementia (Gale et al., 2018). According to a Norwegian study, Alzheimer's disease causes 57% of all dementia cases, followed by vascular dementia (10%), Lewy body dementias (4%), and frontotemporal dementia (2%) (Gjøra et al., 2021). Similar numbers are presented in international studies. It has been estimated that 50 million people worldwide live with of dementia, increasing to approximately 150 million people in 2050.

Dementia diseases have different symptom profiles, displaying the complexity of the dementia syndrome. Dementia caused by Alzheimer's disease is hallmarked with memory loss, language problems, orientation problems, reduced problem-solving capacity, apathy, and depression, and it develops gradually (Scheltens et al., 2016). Vascular dementia is caused by one large or many smaller ischemic or haemorrhagic cerebral strokes. The onset is often more sudden than for patients with Alzheimer's disease, although it can also develop gradually, and impairment in attention, processing, judgement, and executive function is common. Frontotemporal dementia is caused by neurodegeneration in the frontal or the temporal lobes of the brain. The dementia is progressive in its nature, and it is identified by early changes in personality with loss of disinhibition and executive functions. Dementia with Lewy bodies and Parkinson's disease dementia are referred to as Lewy Body Dementias, as they share a common pathology and symptomatology. Typical symptoms for patients with Lewy Body Dementias are impaired visuospatial orientation and reduced executive function, fluctuating attention, visual hallucinations, sleep disturbances, and the typical motor symptoms seen in Parkinson's disease (Gale et al., 2018).

The differences in the presentation of the dementia diseases reflect where in the brain the neurodegeneration or injury is located as well as the pathology causing the neuron loss. As an example, Alzheimer's disease is associated with deposits of amyloid plaques and neurofibrillary tangles in the brain (DeTure & Dickson, 2019), while dementia caused by a stroke or haemorrhage in the brain (vascular dementia) is associated with neuronal loss caused by vascular damage to brain cells. To complicate the picture even more, several patients with dementia have pathology from more than one disease. Studies have found mixed dementia pathology in a waste number of persons with dementias (Rahimi & Kovacs, 2014). Mixed dementia pathologies may complicate the clinical picture of the disease, making the diagnostic work up, treatment, and care difficult. For the person with dementia and their relative, the exact diagnosis may not be very important, as they are more concerned about the symptoms. Symptoms as changes in personality, apathy, irritation, and repetitive behaviour may be of special concern. As the dementia and the symptoms progress, the persons' religious references and meaning in life may change. This will influence on the patient with dementia and its relative. If the person with dementia loss interest in religion, the relative can experience sadness as they cannot longer share the community in taking part in religious activities.

Most of the persons with dementia will experience a progression of their disease, with increased cognitive decline and more severe symptoms. The tempo and course of the disease progression, how, and when the cognitive decline and symptoms appear may be different from person to person. This uniqueness in the individual's presentation of the dementia disease, and the variety in the course of the disease, build up under the complexity of dementia. Although patients with the same dementia disease generally share the same cognitive profile and symptoms, two persons with the same dementia disease may differ in how the disease presents for them. Depending on the type of the dementia and the severity of the disease, the person's insight and ability to describe the symptoms and his/her needs may be impaired. As a result, the healthcare staff's ability to provide adequate care and treatment may be hampered. Each person with dementia should therefore be examined extensively, and they should be offered treatment and care tailored to their symptoms and function.

## Risk factors for dementia

The complexities of the brain and the complexity of the dementia diseases can be seen from the huge range of risk-factors causing dementia. In a Delphi process including many of the world's best dementia researcher, the *2024 Lancet Commission of the dementia prevention, intervention, and care* concluded that 14 modifiable risk factors accounted for around 45% of dementia cases in the world (Livingston et al., 2024). Some risk factors are important in early life (like education), some in midlife (like hearing loss, traumatic brain injury, and hypertension), and some in later life (like smoking and depression). Saying that 55% of the modifiable risk factors are unknown and there are also unmodifiable risk factors like the genes coding for aggregation of pathological proteins in the brain causing Alzheimer's disease (Livingston et al., 2024). The many risk factors for dementia, their complexity, and the interconnection can be both an advantage and a disadvantage for the person with dementia and their relatives. A variety of risk factors give the patient and healthcare staff several possible interventions that alone or in combination could reduce the risk for dementia. As an example, a healthier diet and lifestyle, with less fat, more vegetables, less alcohol, and no smoking may promote better health. However, the complexity and interconnection between risk factors make it difficult to isolate and understand the effect of one intervention. We see that risk factors are found on a group level, but the individual may not avoid dementia despite living healthy. Although several cohort studies have identified risk factors for dementia, it has been difficult to demonstrate the effect of interventions targeting these risk factors (Rakesh et al., 2017). As an example, a Mediterranean diet has in cohort studies been found to be associated with reduced risk of mild cognitive decline and Alzheimer's disease, but trials with Mediterranean diet as an intervention have only found minor effects on episodic- and working memory (Fu et al., 2022). Better effect has been demonstrated for physical exercise, which in trials attenuate cognitive decline in persons with mild cognitive impairment and dementia (Law et al., 2020), and music therapy which has been found to improve the quality of life, cognition, and neuropsychiatric symptoms like depression in persons with dementia (Lin et al., 2023).

## Treatment and care

Treatment and care of dementia is both psychosocial interventions and pharmacological treatment. Person-centred care is the first choice, meaning that the person is in the centre of the treatment, and that the treatment should be individualized and adapted to the person's needs (Kitwood & Bredin, 1992). Person-centred care and existential health are further discussed in Chapter 6 of this book, and I will only describe pharmacological treatment of dementia to chatter more light on the complexity of dementia. Most research has been done on pharmacological treatment for Alzheimer's disease, where two classes of medicines have a moderate effect in slowing down the progression of the disease. Recently, a class of medicines that slow down cognitive declining and prevent amyloid plagues from forming in persons with Alzheimer's disease has been approved by the Food and Drug Administration (FDA) in the USA. They are antibodies that remove the aggregated pathological antibodies in the brain, and they may be a game-changer in dementia treatment if they can prevent or slow down the progression of the disease. The downside of the newly marketed treatment is high costs, a need of early diagnosis and close follow-up during treatment, and potential severe side effects like micro bleedings and inflammations in the brain (Cummings et al., 2023). It has been calculated that the costs for the new medicines, if prescribed to all patients in Europe with the right indication, will be half of the costs for all medicines used in Europe. There is therefore an ongoing discussion whether the medicines should be approved for use in Europe. As dementia is not curable, most pharmacological treatment prescribed to people with dementia would be to reduce symptoms like depression, anxiety, apathy, psychosis, irritation, and aggression. Psychopharmacological treatment like antidepressants, anxiolytics, and antipsychotics is widely described to persons with dementia but the balance between the effect and the side-effects is delicate and complex. Finding the right indication for starting psychopharmacological treatment, evaluating the effect and side-effects of the treatment, and reduce or stop treatment at the right time builds up on the complexity of dementia. Prescribing medicines can also remove the focus from psychosocial interventions, which the persons with dementia, their relatives, and staff of the healthcare service rather support.

Another example of the complexity of psychopharmacological treatment in dementia is treatment of psychotic symptoms in Lewy Body Dementia. Persons with Lewy Body Dementia have low levels of dopamine in their brains, causing symptoms like tremor, bradykinesia (slowness of movement), rigidity, and postural instability (Garcia-Ptacek & Kramberger, 2016). Prescribing levodopa or other medicines that increase the dopamine level will reduce the symptoms. Unfortunately, increased dopamine levels in the brain can cause hallucinations and other psychotic symptoms, which is common in people with Lewy Body Dementia. To treat psychotic symptoms, antipsychotics are usually prescribed which lower the dopamine level in the brain. The effect can be reduced psychotic symptoms, but increased motor symptoms. The person should take part in the discussions before prescribing antipsychotics for psychosis in Lewy Body Dementia, as their opinion is important to decide what is important for them.

## Conclusion and recommendations

In conclusion, dementia is caused by neurodegeneration or injury to the brain. The complexity of the brain is reflected in the range of symptoms of dementia, that several diseases may cause dementia, and in a variety of risk factors associated with dementia. Further, treatment and care of dementia should be person-centred, balancing the effect of the psychosocial intervention or pharmacological treatment to the possible side-effect. The complexity and the plasticity of the brain are an opportunity to increase the persons well-being and quality of care through training, psychosocial interventions and stimulation. Focusing on what is important for each person with dementia is essential and may help the person experience meaning in life. Person-centred care is the goal of treatment and care for person with dementia, and psychosocial interventions should be implemented before mediations are prescribed.

## References

Cummings, J., Apostolova, L., Rabinovici, G. D., Atri, A., Aisen, P., Greenberg, S., Hendrix, S., Selkoe, D., Weiner, M., Petersen, R. C., & Salloway, S. (2023). Lecanemab: Appropriate use recommendations. *J Prev Alzheimers Dis, 10*(3), 362–377. https://doi.org/10.14283/jpad.2023.30

DeTure, M. A., & Dickson, D. W. (2019). The neuropathological diagnosis of Alzheimer's disease. *Mol Neurodegener, 14*(1), 32. https://doi.org/10.1186/s13024-019-0333-5

Fu, J., Tan, L. J., Lee, J. E., & Shin, S. (2022). Association between the mediterranean diet and cognitive health among healthy adults: A systematic review and meta-
analysis. *Front Nutr*, *9*, 946361. https://doi.org/10.3389/fnut.2022.946361

Gale, S. A., Acar, D., & Daffner, K. R. (2018). Dementia. *Am J Med*, *131*(10), 1161–1169.
https://doi.org/10.1016/j.amjmed.2018.01.022

Garcia-Ptacek, S., & Kramberger, M. G. (2016). Parkinson disease and dementia. *J Geriatr
Psychiatry Neurol*, *29*(5), 261–270. https://doi.org/10.1177/0891988716654985

Gjøra, L., Strand, B. H., Bergh, S., Borza, T., Brækhus, A., Engedal, K., Johannessen,
A., Kvello-Alme, M., Krokstad, S., Livingston, G., Matthews, F., Myrstad, C., Skjel-
legrind, H., Thingstad, P., Aakhus, E., Aam, S., & Selbæk, G. (2021). The prevalence
of mild cognitive impairment, dementia, and its subtypes in a population-based sam-
ple of people 70 years and older in Norway: The HUNT Study. *J Alzheimers Dis*,
*79*(3). https://doi.org/10.3233/JAD-201275

Kiss, M. (2020). *Demographic outlook for the European Union 2020.* https://data.
europa.eu/doi/10.2861/999213

Kitwood, T., & Bredin, K. (1992). Towards a theory of dementia care: Personhood and
well-being. *Age Soc*, *12*, 269–287.

Law, C. K., Lam, F. M., Chung, R. C., & Pang, M. Y. (2020). Physical exercise at-
tenuates cognitive decline and reduces behavioural problems in people with mild
cognitive impairment and dementia: A systematic review. *J Physiother*, *66*(1), 9–18.
https://doi.org/10.1016/j.jphys.2019.11.014

Lin, T.-H., Liao, Y.-C., Tam, K.-W., Chan, L., & Hsu, T.-H. (2023). Effects of music
therapy on cognition, quality of life, and neuropsychiatric symptoms of patients with
dementia: A systematic review and meta-analysis of randomized controlled trials.
*Psychiatry Res*, *329*, 115498. https://doi.org/10.1016/j.psychres.2023.115498

Livingston, G., Huntley, J., Liu, K. Y., Costafreda, S. G., Selbæk, G., Alladi, S., Ames,
D., Banerjee, S., Burns, A., Brayne, C., Fox, N. C., Ferri, C. P., Gitlin, L. N., Howard,
R., Kales, H. C., Kivimäki, M., Larson, E. B., Nakasujja, N., Rockwood, K.,…, &
Mukadam, N. (2024). Dementia prevention, intervention, and care: 2024 Report of
the Lancet standing Commission. *The Lancet*, *404*(10452), 572–628. https://doi.
org/10.1016/S0140-6736(24)01296-0

Rahimi, J., & Kovacs, G. G. (2014). Prevalence of mixed pathologies in the aging brain.
*Alzheimer's Res Ther*, *6*(9), 82. https://doi.org/10.1186/s13195-014-0082-1

Rakesh, G., Szabo, S. T., Alexopoulos, G. S., & Zannas, A. S. (2017). Strategies for dementia prevention: Latest evidence and implications. *Ther Adv Chronic Dis*, *8*(8–9),
121–136. https://doi.org/10.1177/2040622317712442

Scheltens, P., Blennow, K., Breteler, M. M., de Strooper, B., Frisoni, G. B., Salloway, S., & Van
der Flier, W. M. (2016). Alzheimer's disease. *Lancet*, *388*(10043), 505–517. https://doi.
org/10.1016/S0140-6736(15)01124-1

# 8 Types of dementia, daily living, and existential health

*Knut Hestad and Knut Engedal*

There are connections between types of dementia and existential health, but this is also influenced by personality, coping strategies, and the person's cultural and religious background and practice. Existential meaning may change in accordance with severity, type of cognitive impairment, and insight in own illness. Nevertheless, it is important for the person to keep a high level of activity and build upon his or her interests from their former way of living, to maintain quality of life when living with dementia.

## Dementia

Dementia comes from the term "dementare", which means that the person who has the condition is de-connected from mental processes. This would indicate that persons with dementia are crazy or mad. This is of course not the situation. In degenerative brain disorders causing dementia, such as Alzheimer's disease, Parkinson's disease, Lewy Body disease, and Fronto-temporal degenerative disorders, to mention the most common ones, we witness a progressive deterioration where various cognitive abilities deteriorate over time. Due to the cognitive decline, dysfunction in activities of daily living (ADL) will arise, leading to dependency on others. During the progression, various changes of behavior will be present such as anxiety, depression, apathy, delusion, hallucination, agitation, and restlessness. There may also be some personality changes especially in patients with more frontotemporal lobe damages.

In most cases, even when the brain disorder progresses to a very severe neurocognitive stage, mental activities will still be preserved, and the diseased person does not completely lose the "self" but the meaning in life will be influenced by severity of cognition, ADL decline, personality changes, behavioral changes, and insight into one's own disease. The core of earlier (before debut of dementia) existential traits due to personality, coping strategies, experiences in lived life, including cultural and spiritual understanding, and belief will to some extent be preserved. Therefore, it is important to know about what made up the content of life for the person, not pieces of it, but at least

DOI: 10.4324/9781003517733-10

enough to connect and have a meaningful talk or discussion with him or her. If you do not know the person, it will be very difficult to have a meaningful conversation.

## Being diagnosed with dementia

Being diagnosed with dementia will probably create an existential crisis and mental reaction in most of us. The perception, thoughts, feelings, and behaviors change. Changes related to living with a dementing disorder will influence mental and existential health and coping strategies. Our personality traits are important for appropriate coping strategies that can help in coping with life-threatening situations. This is why understanding the personality of the patient becomes important when he or she is diagnosed with dementia. However, even though people live with impaired memory functioning, they will know and have a strong feeling of who they are. The dementia must be very severe before they lose this knowledge, and usually it is not lost. This is important for the professional caregivers to know and maintain respect for the patient. This is personalized care, and the sense of meaning in life will often be lost if the autonomy of the patient is threatened.

## The present and past

When talking with patients who are suffering from dementia it may seem like present and past chronology to some extent merge. The perception of time (i.e. timeline) almost dissolves. The focus of their life is not here and now but stories from the life they have lived pop up. What they had for dinner 30 minutes ago may be as present as what happened to them in their childhood 60 or 70 years ago (the former is often forgotten). We call the latter "the present past" which has a significant meaning for making their life today meaningful. It is an unclear chronological reference point for past and present, which more or less is intertwined with each other. The past and present merge, giving their stories a special flavor. The time concept becomes relative. They can talk about their parents as if they were alive and present, even if they themselves were 95 years of age. What the participants often underline as important for them is the relationship with their family. To understand the present person, you need to understand their life story with childhood and midlife.

The merging of past and present underscores the complexity of communication with individuals who have major cognitive impairment and highlights the need for flexibility when communicating with people who have developed dementia. These patients need cues to continue verbal communication.

It is interesting to see and hear when they sing songs from the past, overlearned rhymes and poems that still may be remembered, and that the patients have a good time when they present them. This may be something to use to keep the quality and meaning in life as high as possible. (More about this in Chapters 11 and 14.) To come closer to existential challenges we will proceed to the specific dementia diseases. How does the disease affect the individual? We will concentrate on the most common form of dementia, Alzheimer's disease, but also briefly mention vascular dementia and frontotemporal dementia (cf Chapter 7 in this book).

## Alzheimer's disease

Alzheimer's disease was diagnosed by Alois Alzheimer in the beginning of the 19th century (Beach, 2022; Bermejo-Pareja & Del Ser, 2024). It was based on one patient, Mrs. Auguste Deter, who was 51 years old when diagnosed with the disease. She started to behave irrationally with delusions, hallucinations, and agitation and had memory loss (Alzheimer, 1907). Her brain disease progressed fast. Dr. Alzheimer had the possibility to examine her brain and suggested that plaques outside the neurons and tangles inside the neurons were responsible for the brain disorder. The disease shows a progressive decline and there is so far no cure or vaccines. It probably has a silent development (more than ten years) before it manifests with cognitive impairments, most often with memory deficits. However, occasionally language or visual constructive problems may be the first symptom depending on location of the brain damages (Barnes et al., 2015; Weintraub et al., 2012).

## Dementia of Alzheimer's disease, various severity

In the transition, from "healthy" to manifest symptoms the patient may have substantial existential difficulties, especially after a possible diagnosis of Alzheimer's disease. He or she knows that the disease will progress, with more cognitive difficulties and dependency in ADL functions in the years to come. Often the diseased persons compare their situation with a similar development in their mother, father, or another family member having dementia in a severe stage, being severely dependent in ADL and living in nursing homes. In the first stage of dementia (usually with milder forms of memory impairment) the patient is normally aware of the situation, and in a way their whole existence is in play. This may also be a very difficult situation for the next-of-kin. Alzheimer's disease is a potentially deadly disease and for those of us who are health personnel the question is how we may be able to comfort and bring some kind of hope in this difficult situation.

Some, due to their personality traits and coping strategies, try to do the best out of the situation. They may change their environment to a more suitable place to live, especially if they live alone. Some go to internet and search for training programs that could slow down the progression and start to train both physically and cognitively. They do not want to be a burden for the next-of-kin or other family members. Others are more reluctant to make changes in their daily life, and another type of people tend to be anxious, depressed, and paralyzed. Nevertheless, people behave differently and the questions they ask for themselves and the action they take are different in this early stage of the disease, but all ask questions related to the disorder. What is going to happen to me? Who will take care of me if the disorder progresses and my ability to care for myself becomes worse? Is there any medication that will help? Where am I going to live? Can I still live at home? Do I have to move to a nursing home? Why me? This is unfair! Such questions and statements are often expressed by the diseased.

As the disease progresses, insight into own impairments will decrease, and in a moderate stage of dementia many patients will report good quality of life, as shown in many studies. We here refer to some Norwegian studies (Bruvik et al., 2012; Hvidsten et al., 2018; Mjørud et al., 2014; Rosness et al., 2011). It seems that their perception of own impairment is better compared to the reported quality of life rated by their family members (Bruvik et al., 2012). In interviews with people with moderate dementia, people often report that they enjoy doing activities that they used to perform earlier in life. In many cases this is a fantasy. They do not perform the activities but have a perception of doing it. However, people suffering from co-morbid depression, anxiety, or having psychotic symptoms will not have this positive attitude and perception of their daily life and meaning in life.

At a certain point of progression of the disease, many people with Alzheimer's disease forget that they forget. They may not remember that their husband died just a year ago or identify persons that they meet almost every day. Some do not recognize their husband or children. Their life has changed, and their conception of being in the world has changed. They may not know where they are and why they are here, not even in their own home or in a nursing home. Some have a notion that they are not at home and may ask when they are going to leave 'this hotel' and travel back home. To some degree, they may have the ability to locate where they are, but this knowledge is reduced, which may confuse their perception of who they are and who their next-of-kin are. A possible feeling of loneliness can be there, as the person expresses that no one ever comes to visit, even if relatives are there every week.

In the late stages of dementia of Alzheimer's type, where the patients have difficulties in expressing their meanings and feelings with spoken language, we really do not know exactly how their thoughts are about their existential meaning in life. We must guess by evaluating their behavior on a daily basis. A calm and smiling person with severe dementia, enjoying a good meal and good company may have a good life. A grumpy and agitated person has probably not a good life. In this stage of dementia, the person (who often lives in a nursing home) is dependent on others, also when it comes to existential decisions and even existence. In addition, they may have lost their capacity to understand and give consent to care and treatments, and thus, their decision-making ability is restricted. However, they may still have reflections related to their situation in life and lived life, which should be listened to and be respected. Shared decision-making may be a choice in these situations.

## Alzheimer's disease early in life

There are people who develop dementia of Alzheimer's type as early as 40 or 50 years of age. They are few, less than one percentage of those with Alzheimer's disease. Those who are affected at 45 years of age will necessarily have other existential challenges than those who are 85. These young ones are in the midst of their life and may have a family with children who are adolescents or even younger. In our experience, younger patients react differently to receiving the diagnosis of Alzheimer's disease than older patients. There are so many questions to be answered and challenges to be resolved. What will happen to my family when I am not able to contribute? How will the disease change my relationship with my family? What about the economy for me and my family when I can't work?

## Other forms of dementia

In other types of dementia, the memory for recent events is not lost to the same degree as in Alzheimer's disease.

Cerebral vascular forms of dementia are a result of smaller or bigger strokes. This is the second most experienced form of dementia. Almost every stroke will give some kind of cognitive deficits, but necessarily not so much that they qualify for a dementia diagnosis. However, studies show that the frequency of dementia after stroke varies but is about 30% within 3–12 months after the stroke episode (Leys et al., 2005; Tatemichi et al., 1992).

Often cerebral vascular dementia develops like a staircase you are going down. If the risk factors for more strokes are still present, the patients often develop dementia due to brain damage (Leys et al., 2005). Therefore, it is extremely important to reduce factors that can be related to strokes like being overweight, high blood pressure, high cholesterol, etc.

Some of the very old people with dementia after a stroke, have in addition Alzheimer's disease that becomes visible. Among these patients, we see the same pattern of symptoms as described above with Alzheimer's disease.

The existential threats among people with poststroke dementia (without Alzheimer's) will in many cases be the same as for people with Alzheimer's disease due to the decline in cognition, ADL, and changes in insight and behavior. We have learned from studying stroke patients that these often do not have an overview of their cognitive deficits and are more worried about physiological deficits like toilet functions or motor deficits than their cognitive deficits (Evensen et al., 2024). However, in the long run it is important to pay attention to both physical and cognitive performance. If not, the patient can be isolated, vicious circles may develop, and depression can be a result.

## Frontotemporal lobe dementia is another matter

This type of dementia is due to degeneration of the frontal lobes and partly of the temporal lobes of the brain. The people with this form of dementia are in most cases below the age of 70 years. About one in four have a hereditary disorder. Usually, dementia has an insidious start with a progressive worsening course over many years. In the early stages, we differentiate between two main types, the behavioral type (55%) and the language type (45%). In these early stages, the patients do not fulfill the criteria for dementia, although they have declined cognitively, mainly with impaired executive abilities and impaired insight into their own disabilities. Memory function may be intact, and progression to dementia may take many years. Due to loss of executive function, little empathy, poor social behavior, and poor insight, their perception of meaning in life is changed.

Especially, the persons with the behavioral type and no insight into their own behavior are difficult to care for; "I have no problems", the patients say, lacking insight into their own situation. These patients can be a challenge to interact with for everyone. However, it may be important where in the frontotemporal lobes their biggest damage is. We have seen that damage in the right frontal lobe compared to damages in the left cause more behavioral disturbances, whereas damage in the left frontotemporal region causes language problems (Broca aphasia) and depression. In persons with frontotemporal damage, the downplay of deficits or difficulties are usually very clear. With the focus is more on the left side of the brain; the patients may show substantial depressive symptoms and the feeling that something is wrong with them. Their thoughts are therefore that they must be helped in some way or another. However, patients with frontotemporal dementia most often have damage of both their left and right frontal lobes and therefore show up with behavioral disturbances. Their next-of-kin may need a lot of support seeing that their loved ones develop such a change of behavior.

Personality change may be seen in many types of dementia. It is a complex story related to the person's brain damage. Even if the change in personality may be linked to frontal lobe dementia, it can also be seen in Alzheimer's disease and other forms of dementia, preferably with a different brain damage than in the hippocampus area. Premorbid personality can be important when lack of impulse control due to brain damage manifests. The man with a temper no longer controls his behavior, or the woman who always was kind and never argued and always restrained herself now loose impulse control and all kinds of "dirty" words are expressed. The personality change becomes a problem for the surroundings when it results in aggressive behavior but is also unpleasant when the patient scolds those who are in contact with him or her. For relatives, personality changes can trigger feelings of grief and confusion, and there may be a need for help to understand and navigate the situation, as well as for emotional support.

## How do we meet patients with dementia?

The individual with dementia is usually dependent on care of other people, most often in nursing homes when progressed to a severe stage. Due to the lack of highly educated personnel in dementia care, the main caretaker may be a person with little or no education or experience in dementia care. Thus, the quality of care differs a lot between nursing homes, as well as between wards in the same nursing homes (Kirkevold & Engedal, 2006). The nursing homes are supposed to give "person centered care". If they do so and follow up as good as they can, the person with dementia may have a chance to still be able to live up to existential possibilities even in a very difficult and limited situation for him or her. We may then ask how should the patient/resident be able to have as good existential health as possible? How could we help people with dementia to maintain their autonomy even if they are severely diseased? Referring to the evidenced-based knowledge, dementia care should be provided using person-centered care, which implies that we always should try to understand the behavior of the patient using his or her perspective, to improve their meaning and quality of life.

People are different, and they have lived different lives. A common existential situation is that many people with dementia need cues to remember or act. Nursing home residents with dementia often have a pretty good idea about when they are going to have their meals, but they forget it soon after they have eaten. They probably use the cues in the environment, like when the staff are starting to prepare what is going to take place next. Their behavior changes and the residents' sense and are aware of it.

One can ask how much resources it is worth to use on existential health in the great number of nursing home residents with dementia. Our answer to this is how you would like to be met when you are down and out!

## References

Alzheimer, A. (1907). Uber eigenartige Erkrankung der Hirnrinde. *All Z Psychiatr, 64*, 146–148.

Barnes, J., Dickerson, B. C., Frost, C., Jiskoot, L. C., Wolk, D., & van der Flier, W. M. (2015). Alzheimer's disease first symptoms are age dependent: Evidence from the NACC dataset. *Alzheimers Dement, 11*(11), 1349–1357. https://doi.org/10.1016/j.jalz.2014.12.007

Beach, T. G. (2022). A history of Senile Plaques: From Alzheimer to amyloid imaging. *J Neuropathol Exp Neurol, 81*(6), 387–413. https://doi.org/10.1093/jnen/nlac030

Bermejo-Pareja, F., & Del Ser, T. (2024). Controversial past, splendid present, unpredictable future: A brief review of Alzheimer disease history. *J Clin Med, 13*(2). https://doi.org/10.3390/jcm13020536

Bruvik, F. K., Ulstein, I. D., Ranhoff, A. H., & Engedal, K. (2012). The quality of life of people with dementia and their family carers. *Dement Geriatr Cogn Disord, 34*(1), 7–14. https://doi.org/10.1159/000341584

Evensen, J., Soberg, H. L., Sveen, U., Hestad, K. A., Moore, J. L., & Bronken, B. A. (2024). Individualized goals expressed by patients undergoing stroke rehabilitation: An observational study. *J Rehabil Med, 56*, jrm15305. https://doi.org/10.2340/jrm.v56.15305

Hvidsten, L., Engedal, K., Selbæk, G., Wyller, T. B., Bruvik, F., & Kersten, H. (2018). Quality of life in people with young-onset Alzheimer's dementia and frontotemporal dementia. *Dement Geriatr Cogn Disord, 45*(1–2), 91–104. https://doi.org/10.1159/000487263

Jansen, W. J., Ossenkoppele, R., Knol, D. L., Tijms, B. M., Scheltens, P., Verhey, F. R., Visser, P. J., Aalten, P., Aarsland, D., Alcolea, D., Alexander, M., Almdahl, I. S., Arnold, S. E., Baldeiras, I., Barthel, H., van Berckel, B. N., Bibeau, K., Blennow, K., Brooks, D. J.,…, & Zetterberg, H. (2015). Prevalence of cerebral amyloid pathology in persons without dementia: A meta-analysis. *JAMA, 313*(19), 1924–1938. https://doi.org/10.1001/jama.2015.4668

Kirkevold, O., & Engedal, K. (2006). The quality of care in Norwegian nursing homes. *ScandJCaringSci,20*(2),177–183.https://doi.org/10.1111/j.1471-6712.2006.00396.x

Leys, D., Hénon, H., Mackowiak-Cordoliani, M. A., & Pasquier, F. (2005). Poststroke dementia. *Lancet Neurol, 4*(11), 752–759. https://doi.org/10.1016/s1474-4422(05)70221-0

Mjørud, M., Røsvik, J., Rokstad, A. M., Kirkevold, M., & Engedal, K. (2014). Variables associated with change in quality of life among persons with dementia in nursing homes: A 10 months follow-up study. *PLoS One, 9*(12), e115248. https://doi.org/10.1371/journal.pone.0115248

Rosness, T. A., Mjørud, M., & Engedal, K. (2011). Quality of life and depression in carers of patients with early onset dementia. *Aging Ment Health, 15*(3), 299–306. https://doi.org/10.1080/13607861003713224

Tatemichi, T. K., Desmond, D. W., Mayeux, R., Paik, M., Stern, Y., Sano, M., Remien, R. H., Williams, J. B., Mohr, J. P., Hauser, W. A., et al. (1992). Dementia after stroke: Baseline frequency, risks, and clinical features in a hospitalized cohort. *Neurology, 42*(6), 1185–1193. https://doi.org/10.1212/wnl.42.6.1185

Weintraub, S., Wicklund, A. H., & Salmon, D. P. (2012). The neuropsychological profile of Alzheimer disease. *Cold Spring Harb Perspect Med, 2*(4), a006171. https://doi.org/10.1101/cshperspect.a006171

# 9 Beyond memory loss

## The role of emotion and narrative in dementia care

*Gry Stålsett*

## Introduction

Life narratives are essential in constructing a coherent sense of self and facilitating emotional connections. They help individuals organize fragmented life moments into a unified story, offering a way to understand who they are and their place in the world (McAdams, 2001). This storytelling process is not only about reflecting on the past but also preserving a sense of identity, especially in times of adversity or cognitive decline. For people with dementia, this becomes particularly significant, as memory loss disrupts their ability to recall life events and maintain a coherent narrative, leading to feelings of disorientation and loss of self (Sabat, 2001).

While dementia impairs cognitive memory, emotional experiences, and existential awareness persist (Kitwood, 1997). This article explores how narrative approaches can be adapted for those with dementia, their emotional and existential significance, and how caregivers can support emotional well-being without relying on memory recall.

## Variability, emotional connection, and possibilities

Emotional processing impairments are a hallmark of dementia, yet they manifest differently depending on the type of dementia and its progression. These impairments often fluctuate and are influenced by individual differences. Despite these challenges, research shows that emotional connection is often more possible than expected.

In *Alzheimer's disease (AD)*, emotional processing impairments are closely tied to cognitive decline, particularly memory loss. While early-stage AD patients may retain some emotional experiences, they increasingly struggle with emotional expression and regulation as the disease progresses. Henry et al. (2016) noted that AD patients experience difficulty expressing and managing emotions, particularly in the later stages, when cognitive faculties have deteriorated significantly. Individuals with AD often fail to recognize negative

DOI: 10.4324/9781003517733-11

emotions like sadness or fear, contributing to emotional blunting and social withdrawal (Phillips et al., 2010).

However, despite these cognitive impairments, many AD patients *retain the ability to experience and express positive emotions*. For example, individuals with AD can still express gratitude, joy, or contentment, particularly in familiar and comforting environments. Studies suggest *that emotional connection is possible even in later stages of the disease*, as patients may respond positively to familiar faces, voices, or experiences that evoke emotional memory (O'Brien & Thomas, 2015). This emotional resilience highlights the importance of continuing efforts to engage emotionally with AD patients, even when cognitive impairments seem overwhelming.

In contrast to AD, *frontotemporal dementia (FTD)*, particularly its behavioral variant (bvFTD), affects emotional and social cognition profoundly from the early stages of the disease. FTD is characterized by significant atrophy in the frontal and temporal lobes, which are critical for regulating emotion and social behavior. This leads to emotional blunting, loss of empathy, and socially inappropriate behaviors. Rosen et al. (2006) described how emotional processing in bvFTD patients is often significantly impaired, with individuals struggling to recognize and respond to emotional cues.

Caregivers often find it difficult to engage emotionally with bvFTD patients due to their diminished capacity for empathy and emotional recognition. Balconi et al. (2011) further demonstrated that these individuals face challenges interpreting emotional cues, exacerbating behavioral issues, and making emotional connections seem elusive. However, even in bvFTD, some research *suggests that emotional engagement remains possible* through non-verbal methods, such as music therapy or sensory stimulation, which can bypass cognitive deficits and evoke emotional responses.

*Vascular dementia (VaD)* and *Lewy body dementia (LBD)* each present unique emotional profiles. VaD, caused by restricted blood flow to the brain, often leads to emotional instability, characterized by episodes of crying, irritability, and emotional outbursts. Emotional regulation in VaD can be unpredictable, and individuals may experience heightened sensitivity to their environment, resulting in mood fluctuations that can be challenging for caregivers to manage.

Lewy body dementia (LBD), however, is marked by fluctuating emotional and psychological symptoms. Individuals with LBD often experience mood swings, depression, and anxiety, which can be compounded by hallucinations and delusions. McKeith et al. (2017) emphasized that the emotional and psychological symptoms of LBD are often variable, with periods of emotional clarity alternating with episodes of confusion or emotional volatility.

Despite these emotional challenges, research shows that emotional connection is still possible in VaD and LBD, especially when caregivers focus on creating a stable and comforting environment. The emotional responses of individuals with these types of dementia can fluctuate, but familiar stimuli (e.g. visual, sounds, smell, touch) or even the voice of a friend or family member and the presence of a trusted caregiver can evoke positive emotional reactions, enabling some form of relational engagement.

## Emotions and selfhood continuity

Despite the cognitive impairments caused by dementia, emotional continuity plays a crucial role in preserving a sense of self. Rom Harré's theory of self-hood demonstrates that individuals with Alzheimer's disease actively maintain aspects of their identity through emotional interactions (Hedman et al., 2013). Even as memory deteriorates, emotional responses – as mentioned, those triggered by familiar stimuli – can help preserve a connection to the individual's pre-disease self. The concept of the "embodied self," adds another dimension to this understanding (see Skaalvik, Normann & Norberg, 2016). Even when verbal communication fades, individuals with dementia can non-verbally *express aspects of their identity* through body language, and movements, such as gestures or emotional reactions. While verbal communication often declines, non-verbal emotional communication may persist longer, such as smiling or grimacing. Emotional well-being in caregivers *is equally important, as it deeply influences the emotional reactions* of the person with dementia (Hughes et al., 2014).

## Life narratives and the role of emotions in identity formation

Life narratives, personal stories individuals tell about their lives, are essential to identity formation, they help people make sense of their experiences and maintain emotional connections. Dementia disrupts this process by fragmenting memory and weakening the ability to recall autobiographical events. Sabat (2001) explains that this disruption can challenge individuals with dementia and their families to maintain a shared understanding of the past, leading to emotional disconnection. Narrative approaches, such as reminiscence therapy, help individuals with dementia maintain a sense of self by revisiting personal histories. In the early stages, these methods can preserve cognitive function, enhance self-esteem, and strengthen social bonds (Surr et al., 2016).

However, dementia does not *necessarily* totally erase an "emotional core" – understood as a capacity to feel and respond emotionally even when memory fades. Emotions provide a foundation for subjective experience, offering a kind of felt continuity and meaning as cognitive memory deteriorates, serving as the "heartbeat" of identity. Narrative work, such as life-story sharing or reminiscence therapy, especially in the earlier phases of dementia helps individuals tap into these emotions, enabling them to reaffirm their identity through emotional connections. Even when a *factual* recall is impaired, these emotionally charged stories carry possibilities to evoke through bodily resonances a sense of self, and continuity and still foster engagement with loved ones and caregivers.

## Emotional legacy: gratitude, bitterness, and emotional residues

Even as cognitive faculties decline, emotions tied to life experiences, such as gratitude and bitterness, can persist. Research shows that some individuals with dementia continue to express gratitude, especially in longstanding relationships, despite memory erosion (Pearson, Clarke, & Wolverson, 2022). This emotional continuity reflects the "emotional core" that endures even as cognitive clarity fades, providing emotional resilience.

Conversely, unresolved emotions, such as bitterness or resentment, may resurface and persist, contributing to emotional disturbances. Cohen and Eisdorfer (2001) found that individuals with unresolved emotional conflicts were more likely to express negative emotions, suggesting that dementia can increase vulnerability to these emotional residues.

## Narrative approaches in dementia care: from memory to emotion

As dementia progresses, memory-based approaches have significant limitations and become less effective due to the increasing difficulty in recalling autobiographical memories. Difficulties in accessing specific memories increase, as well as fragmented or inaccurate recall as mixing unrelated memories or creating «false memories» becomes the new «normality». In moderate to severe stages, individuals may no longer recognize family members or recall significant life events, making traditional narrative work emotionally distressing (Surr et al., 2016). Continuing memory-based methods without adaptation can lead to confusion and distress, emphasizing the need to shift from cognitive recall to approaches that engage the remaining emotional capacities of the individual.

### Transition to sensory-based approaches

As dementia progresses and cognitive decline deepens, transitioning from memory-based therapies to sensory-based interventions becomes essential. Sensory adaptations of narrative therapy have shown promise in connecting with individuals who can no longer rely on verbal recall. Sensory stimuli can evoke emotional responses tied to past experiences without requiring *conscious* memory retrieval (Woods et al., 2018). Here are some examples:

- *Sensory cues:* Familiar scents (e.g., perfumes, baking spices) and tastes from one's cultural background evoke emotions tied to home and family.
- *Movement and dance:* Simple dance steps or movements from past routines help reconnect individuals to joyful or familiar physical memories.

– *Tactile engagement:* Textures and materials like fabrics, garden soil, or wood evoke sensory memories tied to work or hobbies.

– *Rhythm and repetition:* Clapping, tapping, or rocking rhythms align with procedural memory, sparking emotions, and memories without verbal recall.

– *Familiar environments:* Recreating familiar settings or using familiar objects (like tools or household items) evokes feelings of home and identity through muscle memory.

– *Creative expression:* Engaging in drawing, painting, or clay work activates body-based memories, letting individuals express emotions tied to their personal history.

These approaches help people reconnect emotionally to their past, fostering identity and well-being even when memory recall is limited.

## Emotional core as a bridge to identity and meaning

For many individuals with dementia, an "emotional core" may serve as an anchor for identity and meaning, as emotional responses to past life events often persist even when factual recall fades. This emotional essence enables caregivers to create meaningful connections by engaging with emotions rather than focusing on precise memories. Swinton (2011) underscores the existential value of emotional presence, advocating for a caregiving approach centered on "being in the moment." This reframing views the person with dementia as someone whose emotional essence continues to reflect their core self, preserving identity even in advanced stages of the condition. Sometimes it becomes too difficult and might be an illusion serving more comfort for the caregiver than the patient. However, it serves a purpose when caregivers continue to affirm the personhood and dignity of individuals with dementia, which aligns with Kitwood's (1997) person-centered care model.

## Integrating the emotional core metaphor in practice

To apply the emotional core concept in dementia care, caregivers can prioritize emotional engagement over factual accuracy, fostering compassionate connections that honor the enduring self within each person. While the "emotional core" approach suggests that emotions preserve identity in advanced dementia, this may not always hold. Conditions like frontotemporal dementia can lead to severe apathy, reducing emotional responses and making it difficult to connect with any "core self." Advanced dementia may also bring personality changes, such as unfamiliar aggression or paranoia, that obscure previous emotional patterns, and some individuals lose recognition of relationships altogether, making emotional connections difficult to sustain.

These exceptions illustrate that the emotional core approach, while valuable, may not universally apply in advanced dementia. Despite this, there are strong arguments for expecting and supporting an emotional essence in individuals with dementia. Focusing on emotional engagement upholds dignity and preserves relationships, enhancing the well-being of both individuals with dementia and their families. This approach respects individuals as more than their cognitive abilities, affirming their right to be seen as whole and valuable.

Belief in an enduring essence can also provide solace to family members, supporting their resilience and mental health through meaningful engagement with their loved ones. At times, caregivers may even be surprised by sudden moments of emotional connection, underscoring the enduring capacity for relational presence, even in advanced stages of the disease.

## Christine Bryden's reflections

Christine Bryden, an influential dementia advocate, author, and speaker from Australia, was diagnosed with early-onset dementia in 1995 at age 46. Since then, she has dedicated her life to raising awareness and challenging misconceptions about dementia. Through her books, including *"Who Will I Be When I Die?"* and *"Dancing with Dementia,"* Bryden shares her personal journey, emphasizing the importance of seeing people with dementia as individuals with feelings, thoughts, and an enduring sense of self.

Bryden underscores the need to maintain emotional and spiritual connections, even as cognitive challenges intensify. She recounts moments of disconnection and frustration but highlights how caregivers can deeply engage on an emotional and spiritual level. She introduces Martin Buber's concept of the I-Thou relationship, describing it as a sacred, spiritual connection that transcends cognitive loss, allowing caregivers and individuals with dementia to share moments of presence and humanity. Even with memory loss, Bryden felt emotionally grounded through the empathy and presence of her caregivers.

Reflecting on the persistence of self-awareness and emotions as cognitive clarity fades, Bryden describes a strong sense of identity – not from memory but through recognition and support from others. Her reflections reveal how emotional and spiritual connections can bridge the gap created by cognitive decline, vividly illustrating how these engagements can sustain personhood in the face of memory loss.

Bryden's insights emphasize the importance of humor, sensory experiences, and emotional engagement in sustaining meaningful connections. While memory fades, the emotional core often remains intact, allowing for moments of connection that transcend cognitive decline. These reflections demonstrate that dementia care must prioritize emotional and spiritual well-being, fostering relationships that honor dignity, humanity, and the individual's capacity for emotional connection.

## Personal reflections on emotional engagement

Caring for a loved one with dementia emphasizes the importance of emotional and sensory engagement. My mother, despite severe memory loss, continues to respond to familiar routines and moments of humor. She often jokes about feeling "like a queen" when being particular about her food. Humor becomes a way for her to express herself and maintain emotional connections. These interactions do not rely on memory recall but allow us to connect through shared laughter and emotional presence.

Research suggests that humor reduces anxiety and fosters emotional connections in dementia care (Spector et al., 2003). It creates a relaxed atmosphere and provides moments of joy, making caregiving feel more relational rather than a set of tasks. In my experience, humor enables emotional clarity between my mother and me, providing comfort and connection.

In the early stages of dementia, my mother expresses what she calls "memory loss grief." She asks our family to become her "co-memory," sharing in the present moments that she can no longer recall on her own. This becomes a shared experience filled with gratitude and joy, which she embraces naturally. She reflects, "I have lost my memory, but I still have my consciousness and presence here and now." On another occasion, she insightfully remarks, "The problem is that memory gives material to what we think, and when my memory fades, it impacts my ability to think long thoughts as before." Her gratitude for my father and her own life remains evident, even as her memory declines, underscoring how deeply emotions and quality of life intertwine, even in the context of cognitive loss.

One powerful experience happens when we visit my mother's cousin, who is also in a dementia ward. Her cousin joyfully declares, "I don't know you, but I do know I love you." Although her cognitive memory is impaired, her emotional memory remains intact, allowing her to recognize and feel love.

Similarly, a colleague of mine recounts a story about a former psychology professor, now suffering from Alzheimer's disease. Her family believes she is "locked in" and unable to recall her past life. However, upon seeing a former colleague, she cries and says, "We know each other, don't we?" Although she cannot recall her professional life, a deep emotional connection emerges. Later, she discusses the meaning of a painting in her room, offering a profound psychoanalytic interpretation, despite having no memory of her profession. Her caregivers are shocked, realizing that beneath the cognitive fog and impairment, her emotional and intellectual essence persists.

Another experience with my mother involves her sudden ability to recall my home, despite her usual inability to remember it. By asking her to "imagine standing on the balcony" and guiding her through the visual memory, she begins to describe it accurately, as if her embodied memory allows her to access images she normally cannot recall. This experience reveals the remarkable and sometimes unexpected ways the brain retains certain forms of memory, and how we can tap into these preserved areas to connect with loved ones.

## Conclusion

In conclusion, despite the cognitive impairments associated with Alzheimer's disease (AD), frontotemporal dementia (FTD), vascular dementia (VaD), or Lewy body dementia (LBD), the concept of an enduring "emotional core" holds profound ethical and existential significance. This emotional essence often persists longer than expected, providing a foundation for connection and identity even as verbal communication fades. The shift from memory-based strategies to emotionally grounded storytelling emphasizes the value of emotional engagement in validating personhood. Sensory-based and non-verbal interventions can tap into emotional memories and enable caregivers to create meaningful interactions, upholding a sense of self and dignity for individuals with dementia.

While emotional responses can vary and are influenced by individual and contextual factors, research supports the potential for caregivers to foster meaningful connections through emotional attunement and awareness of non-verbal cues. This approach can reduce distress and improve the well-being of caregivers and individuals with dementia. However, it is essential to acknowledge that in some cases, such as advanced stages of FTD, severe apathy, or personality changes may limit emotional connections.

Nonetheless, promoting an emotional essence affirms the person's right to be seen as whole and valuable, reinforcing identity even as memory fades. By adopting an emotionally centered caregiving model, we move beyond cognitive limitations and support the emotional and existential essence of those with dementia. This perspective invites a transformative shift in care strategies, enhancing the quality of life for individuals with dementia and the caregivers who support them.

## References

Balconi, M., Bortolotti, A., & Gonzaga, L. (2011). Emotional face recognition, EMG response, and medial prefrontal activity in empathic behaviour. *Neuroscience Research, 71*(3), 251–259.

Cohen, D., & Eisdorfer, C. (2001). *The loss of self: A family resource for the care of Alzheimer's disease and related disorders*. New York: WW Norton & Company

Hedman, R., Hansebo, G., Ternestedt, B. M., Hellström, I., & Norberg, A. (2013). How people with Alzheimer's disease express their sense of self: Analysis using Rom Harré's theory of selfhood. *Dementia, 12*(6), 713–733.

Henry, J. D., Von Hippel, W., Molenberghs, P., Lee, T., & Sachdev, P. S. (2016). Clinical assessment of social cognitive function in neurological disorders. *Nature Reviews Neurology, 12*(1), 28–39.

Hughes, T. B., Black, B. S., Albert, M., Gitlin, L. N., Johnson, D. M., Lyketsos, C. G., & Samus, Q. M. (2014). Correlates of objective and subjective measures of caregiver burden among dementia caregivers: Influence of unmet patient and caregiver dementia-related care needs. *International Psychogeriatrics, 26*(11), 1875–1883.

Beyond memory loss  77

Kitwood, T. (1997). *Dementia reconsidered: The person comes first* (Vol. 20). Buckingham, UK: Open University Press.

McAdams, D. P. (2001). The psychology of life stories. *Review of General Psychology, 5*(2), 100–122.

McKeith, I. G. (2017). Dementia with Lewy bodies: A clinical overview. *Dementia*, 739–749.

O'Brien, J. T., & Thomas, A. (2015). Vascular dementia. *The Lancet, 386*(10004), 1698–1706.

Pearson, M., Clarke, C., & Wolverson, E. (2022). The meaning and experience of gratitude for people living with dementia. *Dementia, 21*(1), 335–352.

Phillips, L. H., Scott, C., Henry, J. D., Mowat, D., & Bell, J. S. (2010). Emotion perception in Alzheimer's disease and mood disorder in old age. *Psychology and Aging, 25*(1), 38.

Rosen, H. J., Wilson, M. R., Schauer, G. F., Allison, S., Gorno-Tempini, M. L., Pace-Savitsky, C.,…, & Miller, B. L. (2006). Neuroanatomical correlates of impaired recognition of emotion in dementia. *Neuropsychologia, 44*(3), 365–373.

Sabat, S. R. (2001). The experience of Alzheimer's disease: Life through a tangled veil. *Psychiatric Bulletin, 27*(1), 39.

Skaalvik, M. W., Normann, H. K., & Norberg, A. (2016). Expressions of sense of self among individuals with Alzheimer's disease. *Research and Theory for Nursing Practice, 30*(2), 161–175.

Spector, A., Thorgrimsen, L., Woods, B. O. B., Royan, L., Davies, S., Butterworth, M., & Orrell, M. (2003). Efficacy of an evidence-based cognitive stimulation therapy programme for people with dementia: Randomised controlled trial. *The British Journal of Psychiatry, 183*(3), 248–254.

Surr, C. A., Smith, S. J., Crossland, J., & Robins, J. (2016). Impact of a person-centred dementia care training programme on hospital staff attitudes, role efficacy and perceptions of caring for people with dementia: A repeated measures study. *International Journal of Nursing Studies, 53*, 144–151.

Swinton, J. (2011). Being in the moment: Developing a contemplative approach to spiritual care with people who have dementia. In A. Jewell (ed.), *Spirituality and Personhood and Dementia*, London: Jessica Kingsley Publishers, 175–185.

Woods, B., O'Philbin, L., Farrell, E. M., Spector, A. E., & Orrell, M. (2018). Reminiscence therapy for dementia. *Cochrane Database of Systematic Reviews* (3), CD001120. https://doi.org/10.1002/14651858.CD001120.pub3.

# Part III

# Existential health in practice

# 10 Existential conversations in dementia

## The card methods

*Peter la Cour, Bendik Sparre Hovet and Trine M. Struer-Tranberg*

It seems to be intuitively true, that old age can lead to an increase in thoughts about existence. When life begins to close its doors, it is natural to think of the life lived, to evaluate it, and maybe regret parts of it. One may have second thoughts about some life choices, about the marriage partner or other significant relationships, about things that might have turned out differently. And the ever-closer ending of life – when can it be welcomed?

This assumption about older age and more existential thoughts is not really supported by research but is often mentioned as a fact (Vaart & Oudenaarden, 2018). There is some evidence that existential thoughts are intensified during illness, especially during serious illness and hospitalization, and some seriously ill hospital patients openly express a need to talk to someone about existential issues (Ausker et al., 2008).

The first mention of a diagnosis of dementia may be just such a period of intensified existential thoughts, even though dementia may not yet be a problematic fact affecting multiple areas of functioning. This might also be the case for the relatives. The future of a progressing disease can be an urgent existential challenge, intensifying the need for existential conversations to clarify what is up and what is down, what is of true value, and what is important to the individual. It is not an easy process to become aware of and explore the individual priorities in life. Are they still the same when living with the disease? Has anything changed? Has anything forced a change?

A search of research articles suggests that this apparent need for existential consideration may not be adequately met, at least by health professionals. A Swedish study concluded that "professionals need training and appropriate qualifications to address existential loneliness related to existential aspects of ageing and care" (Sundström et al., 2019). The care professionals often feel uncomfortable with existential questions. This was the result of a UK study that examined the reasons why the staff *did not* address existential and spiritual issues in palliative care. The staff expressed they had a lack of vocabulary around spiritual (existential) issues, they had personal issues around death and dying, lack of training, fear of not being able to resolve the issues

DOI: 10.4324/9781003517733-13

raised, time constraints, and difficulty in separating spiritual and other needs (Abbas & Dein, 2011).

## Different types of support

Memory changes in dementia affect all types of memory, but not in the same way, as already described in this book. Memory for facts, called *semantic* memory, declines first (for example, remembering the names of politicians, distant cities, etc.). The memory for autobiographical episodes with personal and sensory content (*episodic* memory) declines later (Amieva et al., 2008). This may have practical implications for dementia care. It could be suggested that in the early stages of dementia, the coherent "life story" may be of the greatest value and provide the most meaning as long as it can be grasped as a coherent story in the early stages of dementia. The coherent life story may become less important as dementia progresses. In the moderate stages, lived meaning in the actual, real-life may become more important, and with further progression, recalling episodic memories of meaningful events, relationships, attitudes, and life purposes may be the achievable goal for an existential exchange, as described earlier in this book.

Therefore, any initiative to have existential encounters with people living with dementia may have a different initiation, depending on the degree of progression of dementia and the tastes and preferences of the specific individual.

Below will be described and suggested initiatives for existential encounters in early and mild to moderate stages of dementia as well as their relatives.

## Working with sources of meaning statements

One type of existential exchange between people is talking about what is meaningful in life. As mentioned in Chapter 1, an important and coherent theory about meaning in life has evolved in recent decades. T. Schnell's empirical work on sources of meaning (Schnell, 2020) has led to the development of some semi-structured methods for addressing meaning in life, called the Sources of Meaning Card Methods (SoMCaM) (la Cour & Schnell, 2020). These methods allow an existential conversation to be initiated through cards with statements written on them. The statements encourage and structure an exploratory conversation about the sources of meaning of a person in focus. The statements represent 26 empirically validated sources of meaning covering five domains from which a person may gather meaning in life: *Vertical Selftranscendence,* such as deriving meaning from spirituality or religiosity, *Horizontal Selftranscendence,* such as by trying to make the world a better place, or being connected to nature, *Self-actualization,* deriving meaning in personal development or achievement, *Order,* deriving meaning from structure and predictability, and *Well-being and Relatedness*, deriving meaning from personal relationships or self-care.

The first stage of the method is for the person to read and select the cards they feel most in tune with as an individual. The next step is a semi-structured interview for each selected card in a two-person conversation.

The full 26-card version takes about one hour to complete and requires good cognitive functioning and a good ability to reflect for the person in focus and a partner trained in the conversation structure. It is designed for existential encounters with adults at a time of change in their lives, which could be in the face of serious illness and pain, or it could be related to loss, divorce, or addiction. The method works by providing the framework and questions for the individual to explore their personal sources of meaning, to make them more visible, and to ask for possible changes to make meaningful activities more present in their lived lives.

The full version might be helpful for individuals who have just been diagnosed with dementia and are in the early stages and still able to have a coherent conversation about meaning in life for a longer time. The reason for using a semi-structured method for such a conversation is that such conversations rarely happen by themselves.

The method used in mild dementia does not necessarily aim at getting any precise picture of the sources of meaning, but rather to initiate and explore reflections on the meaning in life, as can be seen in the following case.

## A case from a nursing home

Gry was a woman in her 80s who had been diagnosed with frontotemporal dementia. She lived at a nursing home in Norway. She used to live in her own apartment on the third floor but was unable to live alone without help. Her husband had died of dementia two years ago. She described with horror how different he became, how she lost her life partner a long time before he died. Watching her husband wither away exacerbated Gry's anxiety about her own diagnosis, as she said she "wished they had not told me".

As a study project, two psychology students (Bendik Hovet and Petter Brevik) administered the Sources of Meaning Card Method, followed by a qualitative interview the following week. The intervention and the interview were recorded, transcribed, and treated according to consensus guidelines for qualitative research: Important parts of the verbal exchange were coded and grouped into content themes.

Gry talked about statements that contained four of the five dimensions of meaning, and the cards functioned as what can be called an *existential mirror*. Gry focused on the existential themes the cards evoked in her. The card referring to "horizontal transcendence" Gry associated with the fear she felt of not being able to feel at peace due to the progression of dementia. Prompted by a statement associated with "order and structure", Gry talked about how she felt she lacked the *initiative* to do what she wanted to do. The experience of losing her initiative was what the card meant for her. Other cards also were associated with the loss of initiative, especially to knit and take walks in nature, and they brought up Gry's frustration about feeling trapped within herself. This frustration brought back memories of the smell of resin from her own youth. Her father had given her the task of finding resin, and she could still remember the smell.

The focus on having lost initiative was connected to feelings of *loss and emptiness*. Gry had lost her husband and her home, and now she feared that she would lose herself to dementia. At the start of the intervention, she rejected a card associated with achievement due to feeling empty and lacking initiative, so she felt she was no longer able to achieve anything at all.

Gry's loss was the loss of *agency*. In her words, she no longer had any initiative. She liked to knit and sorely missed knitting again. Everything she needed for knitting was beside her chair in her room. Yet, she was not able to pick up the yarn or the knitting needles. "I'm thinking a lot about it… but I'm not able to do it! Just think about it… everything has stopped for me".

For Gry, the conversation around the cards was overwhelming but also meaningful. She said she would not be able to recall all the fond memories without the conversation. She particularly appreciated that it felt natural and safe to open up about these topics.

After the card intervention, something new happened. While Gry was still frustrated about not being able to knit, she had found another form of agency. In the follow-up interview the next week, Gry told that she had dared to do something she had never done in years. During an evening at the nursing home, listening to a Swedish dance band, she asked one of the men to dance with her. He accepted, and they danced the evening away. She described it as a triumph, clearly excited, and looking forward to doing it again. "I missed it… very much… I enjoyed very much to dance".

No one really knows, but the conversation might have helped her to be more able to dare to engage with life by daring to invite another to dance with her. The conversation might have facilitated the exploration of meaning in life beyond the interview. Talking about meaning with people with dementia may also be important because it implicitly says that life is not over, it is still possible to find meaning.

### Development of a card method for the cognitively impaired

For a person living with a little more progressed dementia or other cognitive challenges, having coherent existential conversations about meaning can be difficult due to cognitive impairment, lack of concentration or drowsiness, as well as time constraints. A simpler version of the card method, aimed at people with mild to moderate cognitive impairment, called the The SoMCaM-7, has been developed to provide for the benefits of an actual conversation about meaning, made accessible and supported by visual prompts, while compensating for the constraints and barriers that can make such a conversation difficult.

The method consists of only seven cards with statements about possible meaning in life, a suggested, lighter structure, and two cards with statements of lived meaningfulness and crisis of meaning.

A manual for use by the interviewer/therapist has been developed to support the conversation. The manual consists of two sets of introductions to the method: one for the person in focus and one for the interviewer/therapist, with instructions on how to use the cards, including prompting questions and the order in which cards are administered.

Using the manual, the interviewer briefly introduces the person in focus to the theme of meaning in life, explains the focus on sources of meaning and what sources of meaning entail, and sets a time frame for the conversation, usually between 30 and 45 minutes. The person in focus is encouraged to talk freely, without regard to what they think should be important, or might be important to others, but rather talk from their own point of view.

The statements on the cards are, for example: "I need to be around other people" or "People should not question the tried and tested". Starting with the five sources of meaning statements, one card at a time is presented to the person in focus, read aloud by the interviewer, and the question 'What do you think about this sentence?' is asked, opening up an exploratory conversation led by the person in focus, and supported by the interviewer.

When a card has been discussed, it should remain visible on the table, and the next card should be presented so that all five cards are visible at the end. This is followed by a simultaneous presentation of the *meaningfulness* and *crisis of meaning* statement cards (Statements: "I live a full life" and "My life seems meaningless"), and again, the person in focus is asked, 'What do you think about these two statements?' When all seven cards have been discussed, the client is asked if they can pick one or two cards that are particularly meaningful for them. Once this has been done, the conversation focuses on the chosen source of meaning cards, why they are of special importance, and how the person in focus eventually could make any small changes in their daily life to make this source of meaning more prominent.

A project to adjust and validate the seven-card method was carried out by Trine Maria Struer-Tranberg at the Specialised Palliative Care Unit at Rigshospitalet, Denmark. The interviewers were nurses who had been trained in both the full and abbreviated versions.

All of the patients were able to complete the full interview and found it useful and rewarding. The cards were helpful in terms of providing a structure to conversations about existential issues, as well as providing visual cues to bring the conversation back on track when focus or concentration was compromised. The open-ended questions about how patients interpreted the cards meant that the conversation could feel tailored to them. One patient described the feeling that the cards had been handpicked for him:

> I thought it was really good to come back to two of the cards after we had talked through all the cards. And I actually thought that it was quite good that you picked those two cards for me; I do not know how you normally pick cards; maybe it is based on how people talk, but you actually picked the two cards that were most important to me.

The interviewing nurses also found the method a useful tool to support existential conversations in terms of removing biases or preconceptions about what should be of importance to the person in focus, supporting persons in telling their life stories and encouraging attention to the person's individual needs.

> I think that because it is structured through cards, it allows you to, well, that it gives a bit of structure to the conversation, yet you get an incredible amount of information about the patient, or the person you sit across. Because for every card is told, you've told a bit of life story. Very quickly you get an insight into another person's life.

Structuring and exploring meaning not only allowed clients to focus their energy on areas of their lives that were high in meaning but also allowed them to find alternatives when faced with limitations:

> Yes, like if you can't go to Spain, which is the biggest wish of my patient at the moment, how can we find something else that could potentially meet a wish to escape the daily routine.

The description, instructions, and printable cards to the Seven-Card Method (SoMCaM-7) are available for full download in several languages at http://somecam.org/card-method-palliative-dementia/.

Future revisions and new language versions will also be available for full download there.

## Discussion

Previously, there have been a few constructive efforts to address existential issues among the elderly reported in research. The 'life story' narrative movement in dementia care has been around for at least 15 years (Mckeown et al., 2010), largely driven by nurses, but it has been of limited use due to too few staff members trained in the procedures (Gridley et al., 2018). A number of self-management life story 'memory books' have been published, and although research on the method is limited, they seem to enhance communication between persons with dementia, relatives, care staff, and residents (Subramaniam et al., 2023).

Apart from the life story-telling movement, only little is known about initiatives for existential talks and support in dementia. In the Netherlands, a project with "Alzheimer cafés" has been implemented (Cuijpers & Van Lente, 2015). People with dementia and their relatives talked about a fixed sequence of topics, including existential themes in a café-like environment. The project was about supporting early diagnostic processes, but it seems like just one project, not an ongoing activity.

Recently, another Dutch group has developed a framework of five themes called the "diamond framework" to help professionals provide existential support. Only a pilot study has been made to evaluate the initiative (Haufe et al., 2024). It concluded that the framework can be used for mild to moderate dementia and relatives. The rationale for the study was the same as in this chapter: the notion that professionals and relatives may be unaware of, or uncertain of, how support can be given on existential issues and reflections.

## Practical implications

In light of the above, the described semi-structured methods for making meanings in life visible through verbal conversation could be suggested for further cautious use in mild (and moderate) dementia. It shall be noted that the methods might be of no meaning or even harmful for people with severe dementia or with no impulse to talk about existential matters. It is also important to stress what is emphasized in the instructions for the seven-card method: whenever the person in focus wants to go somewhere else in the conversation, go with them if it makes sense, and do not stick to the method. The card method is a helping tool for conversation, not an end in itself.

However, it can also be suggested that working with sources of meaning can be a gain for the carers themselves, whether professionals or relatives; help and inspiration to be aware of and not to lose their own sense of meaning in caring for the people living with dementia.

## References

Abbas, S. Q., & Dein, S. (2011). The difficulties assessing spiritual distress in palliative care patients: A qualitative study. *Mental Health, Religion & Culture, 14*(3–4), 341–352.

Amieva, H., Le Goff, M., Millet, X., Orgogozo, J. M., Pérès, K., Barberger-Gateau, P., Jacqmin-Gadda, H., & Dartigues, J. F. (2008). Prodromal Alzheimer's disease: Successive emergence of the clinical symptoms. *Annals of Neurology, 64*(5), 492–498. https://doi.org/10.1002/ANA.21509

Ausker, N., la Cour, P., Busch, C., Nabe-Nielsen, H., & Mørk Pedersen, L. (2008). Danske hospitalspatienter intensiverer eksistentielle tanker og religiøst liv (in Danish). (Danish hospital patients intensifies their existential thoughts and religious life). *Ugeskrift for Læger, 170*(21), 1828–1833.

Cuijpers, Y., & Van Lente, H. (2015). Early diagnostics and Alzheimer's disease: Beyond 'cure'and "care." *Technological Forecasting and Social Change, 93*, 54–67. https://www.sciencedirect.com/science/article/pii/S0040162514000985

Gridley, K., Birks, Y., & Parker, G. (2018). Exploring good practice in life story work with people with dementia: The findings of a qualitative study looking at the multiple views of stakeholders. *Dementia, 19*(2), 182–194. https://doi.org/10.1177/1471301218768921

Haufe, M., Teunissen, S., & Leget, C. (2024). How to provide existential and spiritual support to people with mild to moderate dementia and their loved ones. A pilot study. *PLoS One*, 19(3 March). https://doi.org/10.1371/journal.pone.0298783

Mckeown, J., Clarke, A., Ingleton, C., Ryan, T., & Repper, J. (2010). The use of life story work with people with dementia to enhance person-centred care. *International Journal of Older People Nursing, 5*(2), 148–158. https://doi.org/10.1111/J.1748-3743.2010.00219.X

Schnell, T. (2020). *Psychology of meaning in life*. London and New York: Routledge.

Subramaniam, P., Thillainathan, P., Amirah, N., Ghani, M., & Sharmaid, S. (2023). Life Story Book to enhance communication in persons with dementia: A systematic review of reviews. *PLoS One*, 18(10 October). https://doi.org/10.1371/journal.pone.0291620

Sundström, M., Blomqvist, K., Edberg, A. K., & Rämgård, M. (2019). The context of care matters: Older people's existential loneliness from the perspective of healthcare professionals—A multiple case study. *International Journal of Older People Nursing, 14*(3). https://doi.org/10.1111/opn.12234

Vaart, W., & Oudenaarden, R. (2018). The practice of dealing with existential questions in long-term elderly care. *International Journal of Qualitative Studies on Health and Well-Being, 13*(1). https://doi.org/10.1080/17482631.2018.1508197

# 11 Conversations on existential themes with persons with dementia

*Silje Mathea Nylund*
*and Ingvild Hjorth Feiring*

## Introduction

Conversations about meaning in life may benefit persons with dementia by enhancing their emotional well-being, preserving their identity, and promoting dignity. In a nursing home context, they aid caregivers by facilitating a deeper connection and understanding of the residents, improving the quality of care. They can also support family members by fostering connection, and advocate for compassionate dementia care. In short, these conversations are relevant to anyone who seeks to support individuals with dementia in maintaining a sense of personhood and dignity through the progression of their condition.

Discussing the meaning in life can be challenging due to its abstract nature. It may be easier to talk about what we know about meaning in life and its components, which requires some knowledge on the field. Topics like significance, coherence, orientation, and belonging can be explored, along with sources of meaning like religion and generativity, and the concept of experiencing life as frustratingly empty (crisis of meaning) (Schnell, 2021).

This chapter aims to provide examples to understand experiences of meaning in life for long-term care nursing home residents with dementia, based on theory. We hope that this chapter can be helpful in guiding healthcare professionals, caregivers, and relatives in how to engage in conversations about meaning in life. Although this chapter is mainly aimed at healthcare professionals, these conversations can also be helpful for family members and other caregivers. We have utilised our research as a foundation because there is limited existing work in this area. Our experiences from interviewing residents with dementia living in a long-term care nursing home give us a basis for discussing meaning in life and challenges in conversations about existential topics with these residents. Conversations about meaning in life can give healthcare professionals a better understanding of the person and what matters most to them and further to be able to facilitate a more person-centred care as described in Chapter 9 by Bjørn Lichtwarck.

DOI: 10.4324/9781003517733-14

## Our research: an interview-based study with residents living in long-term care nursing homes

The purpose of the study was to explore the experience of meaning in life for residents with dementia. All residents included were diagnosed with dementia ranging from mild to severe, and they were aged 70 years and older. We conducted ten qualitative semi-structured interviews with nine women and one man, and the interviews were conducted in the residents' private room. The interviews lasted for one to two hours. Their closest relatives were informed and both verbal and written consent was obtained from each resident. Elements from the Meaning and Purpose Scale (MAPS) (Schnell & Danbolt, 2023) were used as a theoretical basis to form an interview guide, with some example questions: "Do you find your life meaningful?", and "how would you describe your life today?".

Residents who contributed to our study showed the ability to understand our questions and create responses about meaning in life despite their diagnosis. They drew on their experiences and memories that represent meaningfulness and sources of meaning. Some provided short answers, others longer stories that were hard to follow. Some required careful guidance and reminding of the topic and questions at hand. This requires curiosity and an openness to listen and explore their narratives although somewhat fractured or hard to understand. What used to be important to them, and what is important to them now? What and who do they miss? What do they find meaningful?

In conversations with nursing home residents, we would first of all focus on equality and avoiding a "patient versus caregiver" dynamic. It is helpful to see each other equally as human beings and connect with the residents on a human level. To discuss these topics, one prerequisite is for the person with dementia to feel safe and be in a secure environment. The conversation itself can be a safe space for a connection between the conversation partners and a deeper understanding of the person with dementia and what they strive for.

We will illustrate a few important issues based on our experiences from the interview study.

## Conversational challenges

Dementia is associated with numerous communication challenges, particularly concerning abstract and existential topics (American Psychiatric Association [APA], 2013; World Health Organization [WHO], 2004). Some people with dementia may give short answers, while others have many associations and may need to be guided back to the topic.

**Case**

Oscar has a severe degree of dementia. He often replies with a «yes» or «no», or spends time seemingly looking for the right words to express himself. Oscar uses few words in parts of the interview.

*S:* Do you find your life meaningful?

*O:* Yes, in certain instances, it is.

*S:* Yes, in what instances is that?

*O:* Well, let's see what it is… For example, it could be something I've learned from my grandparents, and that I've passed on to my grandchildren and so on.

*S:* Yes, that you've learned something from your family that you've passed on?

*O:* Yes.

In this example, we can see that with help Oscar is able to elaborate more. In asking him to elaborate with examples or rephrasing his answers, and being curious, we finally gained a deeper understanding of what was important to him. He emphasised that he missed his family and wanted to return to life as it was before moving to the nursing home, and that he wanted to pass on his knowledge to others. He also said it was difficult to get in touch with others to have a conversation, although he tried.

In doing this, we can understand what is important to him in order to facilitate and possibly increase his sense of belonging and significance. Such conversations may contribute to strengthening the person's feelings of coherence and belonging. It also leads to a better understanding of what matters most to the person with dementia.

### Recommendations

In the following text is some advice for when you encounter challenges in the conversation. You should recognise your role as a conversational partner by reflecting on how cognitive functions differ between you and the resident. Help compensate for cognitive impairment by being curious, collaborative, and facilitating the conversation rather than assuming or directing. Focus on following the resident's lead and gently guiding when needed, such as explaining certain words and concepts. Elaborate with examples, e.g. by asking "Could you tell me some more?" or "Can you give me an example?" Rephrase the question. Paraphrase their answer and ask them to tell you some more. Guide them back to the topic and repeat the questions. Explain concepts that are difficult to understand by using synonyms or gestures.

## "A present past"

The repetition of stories is a common phenomenon for residents with dementia and is often dismissed as a sign of cognitive decline. Staying "in the present" can be difficult.

### Case

Daisy has lived in the nursing home for a year. She has severe dementia. She never gives direct answers to questions about meaning in life. Rather, she goes back in time and brings out examples from growing up, referring to her family and stating that she had a "good upbringing" having everything she needed and parents who cared for her. It is difficult to follow her, and she repeatedly returns to the same memories.

In this conversation, we experienced that Daisy's past played an important role in her present life. We can interpret this as an expression of meaning or an attempt to preserve meaning. In the conversations with Daisy, the timeline was dissolved, drawing meaning from the life she has lived. This could have implications for how Daisy experiences meaning in the present, and how we understand her and the repetition of stories.

### Recommendations

We can help the resident by guiding them back to the present by, for example, asking them how they would describe their life today. Also being aware of how stories and descriptions of situations and experiences in their life can give meaning to the present and in the context of their lifespan.

## Existential themes in nursing homes

Existential themes are fundamental in all life spans and contexts, including end of life and nursing homes. For example, moving to a nursing home can be experienced as an existential challenge in itself as it can lead to isolation and loneliness (Clare et al., 2008; Heggestad et al., 2013). In addition, residents may have experienced several losses that may have great influence on their sense of integrity.

This is why it is so important in nursing homes to be met on a human level. It is crucial to be recognised as a human being with all it entails and how the resident experiences their life now in the context of the nursing home setting.

### Case

Jenny recently moved to the nursing home. She has a mild degree of dementia. She emphasises the importance of being part of a community.

She speaks of the other residents as <u>sick</u> and does not identify with their way of being. "They just sit there and do nothing". She repeatedly states that she is going home and misses her family.

In this example, Jenny refers to the experience of moving away from her home and family, while not feeling at home in the nursing home. She also expressed fear and grief after being diagnosed with Alzheimer's disease, and distanced herself from the other residents. This can be interpreted as a threat to her experience of belonging and connection in that she is separated from her home and herself.

One practical challenge is that these conversations require time, something which is often lacking for healthcare professionals in nursing homes. Setting aside time to focus on meaning in life can be helpful. This is especially important when residents experience the upheaval of moving from their homes to an institution, far from their home environment, family, and the freedom to do what matters most to them.

### *Recommendations*

When you talk about meaning in life, you should always be sensitive to reactions that may arise during and after the conversation. It is important that you provide emotional support and comfort when needed and that you are respectful, empathetic, and give residents the time they need.

### The role of healthcare professionals

Having a conversation about meaning in life with a person with dementia is challenging. To aid healthcare professionals in doing this, we argue that it is helpful to also put emphasis on yourself and what you bring to the conversation. Here are some "reflection tasks" to help becoming aware and navigate your own assumptions about this topic in the context of a nursing home.

### *Recommendations*

We suggest that you take some time to reflect on your own thoughts around meaning in life and what you assume about the experience of a resident with dementia. Do you hesitate to talk about existential topics with people with dementia? What are your thoughts on a resident with dementia's ability to participate in a conversation about existential themes? Are you comfortable broaching this topic, and if not, why? Are you finding it hard to put into words, or have little experience talking about it in general? What is your experience in talking about meaning in life?

Some healthcare professionals are sceptical and resistant to talk about these topics. This scepticism may stem from the belief that it is too difficult for the resident to understand or express themselves as the disease progresses. It may also stem from the belief that the topic is too sensitive for individuals in the final stages of life who live in nursing homes and have been diagnosed with a severe illness. It is natural to hesitate and feel resistance. However, we hope that through conversations like these, you will experience that it is possible and that it provides insight and, in our experience, valuable conversations.

## Final recommendations

Although we argue the benefits of bringing existential topics into the nursing homes, we also need to be cautious when discussing these topics. They may evoke strong emotions and discomfort in residents that are difficult to handle without certain training. And while it is important to respect the potential impact of these conversations, we encourage you to also consider the value it can bring.

Healthcare professionals should set aside some time to talk to residents about the meaning of life. It is helpful as a way to understand what is important to each resident so that we can facilitate sources of meaning and a meaningful daily life. The conversation itself can be meaningful, in that it can create a safe space for sharing and the opportunity for connection. It also creates space for meeting the resident living with dementia as a person with an awareness of their being and sharing a sense of humanity. It can promote the feeling that life still holds significance and that one is significant. It can provide an opportunity for emotional support and comfort. We can get to know the residents' interests through these conversations, allowing us to create individually tailored care plans, which is central to person-centred care. We meet the residents where they are, and from there we can engage them and avoid passivity. Finally, establishing existential contact early in the course of the disease is recommended to provide the best possible person-centred existential care, which can also be important as dementia progresses.

## Example questions

1  How would you describe your life now?
2  What do you care about the most?
3  What is most important to you?
4  What role does religion play in your life?
5  Can you tell us about some important people in your life?
6  What does it take for you to have a good day?
7  What could make your life better?

In conclusion, cognitive impairment or dementia does not exclude the ability to discuss an existential topic. Despite challenges, many people with dementia can elaborate and articulate their experiences and talk about an abstract phenomenon, despite their illness. It is important to do this in the early phases of dementia, even though, in our experience, it is possible to have these conversations in the later stages of the disease. To be "in the present" can be difficult. Orient back to the present but also understand how stories and descriptions of situations and experiences in their life can give an understanding of what is meaningful in the present, and in the context of their lifespan. The presence of the past can have an impact on the experience of meaning in the present for people with dementia. Remember that they should always have the authority to their own experience. Be aware of your own role, adopt an exploratory attitude, and focus on collaboration and equality. We face many challenges, and it's complex – but it is important to try. It is important to have knowledge about the topic and to become confident in discussing it. Most importantly you should respect that it can awaken feelings and reactions that we must follow up on.

## References

American Psychiatric Association (APA) (2013). Diagnostic and statistical manual of mental disorders (5th ed.). American Psychiatric Association. https://doi.org/10.1176/appi.books.9780890425596

Clare, L., Rowlands, J., Bruce, E., Surr, C., & Downs, M. (2008). The experience of living with dementia in residential care: An interpretative phenomenological analysis. *The Gerontologist, 48*(6), 711–720.

Heggestad, A. K., Nortvedt, P., & Slettebø, Å. (2013). The importance of moral sensitivity when including persons with dementia in qualitative research. *Nursing Ethics, 20*(1), 30–40.

Schnell, T. (2021). *The psychology of meaning in life*. Routledge.

Schnell, T., & Danbolt, L. J. (2023). The Meaning and Purpose Scales (MAPS): Development and multi-study validation of short measures of meaningfulness, crisis of meaning, and sources of purpose. *BMC Psychology, 11*(1), 304.

World Health Organization (WHO) (2004). *ICD-10: International statistical classification of diseases and related health problems.* tenth revision, 2nd ed. World Health Organization. https://iris.who.int/handle/10665/42980.

# 12 Navigating dementia with cultural and spiritual sensitivity

## The role of family and caregivers

*Gry Stålsett, Shahram Shaygani, Lars Lien and Lars Johan Danbolt*

### Introduction

Incorporating an understanding of culture, religiosity, and existential needs in dementia care enhances the quality of life for individuals experiencing cognitive decline. Culture and spirituality often form the core of identity and meaning, helping patients retain a sense of self and dignity even as cognitive abilities fade. For patients and families alike, dementia raises profound existential questions, underscoring the need for a compassionate, culturally informed approach.

### Involving families and understanding individual backgrounds

Families are invaluable partners in dementia care, providing insights into the patient's spiritual and cultural values that enable caregivers to shape respectful, personalized care practices. Family members play a critical role in selecting rituals, routines, or traditions that bring comfort and continuity, supporting the patient's sense of identity. As patients may increasingly struggle to communicate their needs, family involvement preserves cherished memories and values (Swinton, 2017). Dementia care can be challenging for families who experience both emotional and practical burdens. Providing support—through counselling, support groups, and spiritual guidance—helps families navigate grief and loss, empowering them to engage more fully in caregiving.

Understanding that emotions are culturally embedded and informed by family contexts, religiosity, and worldview is crucial in dementia care (Tsai et al., 2013). Recognizing these influences allows caregivers to respond empathetically and effectively to patients' emotional needs, fostering a care environment that respects cultural and spiritual identity (Sabat, 2001).

DOI: 10.4324/9781003517733-15

## Spiritual and cultural beliefs in dementia care

Spirituality and religious beliefs can provide emotional comfort, hope, and meaning to elderly people, especially in challenging health situations like dementia (Kevern, 2015). Integrating spiritual or worldview practices—such as meditation or prayer, nature experiences, or use of symbols, music, and texts—enables patients to connect with their faith or orientation systems, bringing stability and reassurance as they cope with cognitive decline (Swift, 2024). Spirituality is an anchor for identity, even when memory and cognition are affected (Swinton, 2017). By incorporating spiritual cultural, worldview-related, and spiritual perspectives into care routines, caregivers support patients' in their ongoing search for a sense of self and connection to something larger.

Cultural awareness also shapes care practices, from daily interactions to dietary preferences and family involvement. Recognizing cultural factors helps caregivers respect patient values, create a familiar environment, and promote engagement. As shown by Oyebode and Parveen (2019), culturally tailored interventions improve emotional well-being, allowing patients to feel seen and respected. For instance, Yoon and Lee (2018) found that cultural values shape caregiving roles significantly in Asian American families. Respecting these values promotes a patient-centered approach. It honors heritage and provides a sense of belonging.

For many patients, dementia can evoke a sense of feeling lost or disconnected from their identity. Care practices that support spiritual and cultural identities offer grounding in times of confusion, helping patients reconnect with core values. Rituals like lighting candles, sharing family stories and pictures, and honoring cultural traditions provide comfort and stability. This helps patients to maintain dignity and self-respect despite cognitive challenges. Culturally sensitive care enhances patient trust and engagement, promoting a positive care experience (Oyebode & Parveen, 2019). An existential approach to caregiver training emphasizes empathy and compassion, encouraging caregivers to see patients as individuals with meaningful life histories and needs.

## Biases, discrimination, and gender issues

Drawing attention to biases, discrimination, systemic racism, and gender dynamics is essential when addressing culture and religiosity in dementia care, as these factors directly impact the depth and respectfulness with which caregivers attend to the religious and cultural dimensions of patient care. When caregivers hold unexamined biases or work within healthcare systems that undervalue the role of culture and spirituality, there is a real risk of neglecting vital aspects of a patient's identity and emotional well-being.

Cultural traditions and spirituality are not merely additions to care; they are often deeply interwoven with a patient's sense of self, emotional stability, and coping mechanisms, particularly in the vulnerable stages of cognitive decline. Caregivers, especially those from minority backgrounds, frequently face discrimination from both patients and colleagues in multicultural settings, leading to feelings of marginalization, burnout, and decreased job satisfaction. Addressing these challenges requires training encouraging caregivers to recognize and mitigate their cultural biases and avoid imposing personal values on patients. Supervision and workplace support can be instrumental in helping caregivers identify unconscious biases that may shape patient interactions, ensuring care is delivered without prejudice based on ethnicity, socioeconomic status, or language abilities. Language barriers further complicate these dynamics, particularly for non-native-speaking caregivers who may struggle with effective communication. Paralikar et al. (2020) emphasize the importance of interpretation services and language support to maintain respectful and culturally sensitive care. Gender roles significantly influence dementia caregiving, often with strong expectations in religious and ethnic minority communities where responsibilities typically fall on women—usually daughters or daughters-in-law—resulting in emotional and physical burdens that can lead to burnout. As more men take on caregiving, especially for spouses, providing adequate support and training is needed to help reduce isolation and alleviate emotional strain and practical helplessness (Robinson et al., 2014).

Dementia care research and practices often reflect a white-centric perspective, favoring Western medical models and overlooking the cultural and spiritual dimensions vital to ethnic minority groups (Zubair, 2023). Training healthcare professionals to address their biases and emotional responses, alongside structural efforts to combat systemic racism, is crucial for fostering an inclusive care environment. Raising awareness about the impact of whiteness and racism in dementia care is essential to providing equitable, culturally sensitive care that truly meets the needs of diverse populations.

## Cross-cultural dynamics in dementia care: balancing tradition, family, and support systems

Dementia care across cultures reveals how cultural values, family roles, and social expectations deeply shape caregiving. To meet the needs of diverse communities, dementia care practices must be culturally sensitive and adaptable. In many cultures, caregiving is primarily seen as a family responsibility, rooted in respect for elders and the belief in familial duty. This can make decisions to seek outside or institutional care challenging, as family members often feel moral or cultural pressure to provide care at home, even when it is physically and emotionally demanding.

Public policy significantly affects family caregiving. Governmental support, including financial aid and respite care, can ease these challenges;

however, policies that overlook cultural nuances often fail to provide effective support in multicultural societies. In some communities, traditional values like filial piety make caregiving an expected responsibility of adult children, while in others, religious beliefs reinforce the idea of home-based care, often at a cost to the caregiver's well-being. Cultural expectations can, therefore, create barriers to seeking outside support, even when institutional care could benefit both the caregiver and the person with dementia.

In immigrant communities, traditional caregiving values may clash with new norms in their adopted countries, leading to emotional strain and underscoring the need for culturally tailored support. Such caregiving often requires a balance between honoring cultural expectations and adapting to new caregiving models. Additionally, perceptions of dementia are influenced by cultural beliefs; some cultures view dementia as a natural part of aging, which can affect decisions around seeking medical intervention or institutional care. Effective dementia care respects these cultural perspectives, offering a sensitive, individualized approach.

In many parts of Asia, for example, caregiving is deeply embedded in family expectations. Yet, urbanization and modernization are straining traditional support structures, making it harder for families to uphold these roles. Ultimately, a cross-cultural approach to dementia care that understands family dynamics, societal expectations, and policy implications is essential for creating respectful and supportive care programs tailored to different cultural contexts.

## Building trust to alleviate existential and spiritual distress in culturally sensitive dementia care

Dementia patients often face existential and spiritual distress, grappling with the loss of identity, isolation, and the search for life's meaning. Addressing these challenges requires a culturally sensitive approach that acknowledges the deep personal and cultural dimensions of these experiences. Existential distress arises as patients confront memory and cognitive loss, leading to feelings of disconnection from their former selves. Spiritual distress may surface alongside, as patients struggle to reconcile their condition with their beliefs and values, which vary significantly across cultural and religious backgrounds.

Emotional regulation strategies are vital for helping patients and caregivers manage these challenges. One approach is incorporating religious and cultural rituals such as prayer, lighting candles, or sharing culturally significant foods—which can help patients maintain a sense of continuity with their faith and cultural identity. These rituals offer emotional solace, grounding patients in familiar practices and providing comfort amid cognitive decline. Integrating such rituals into daily care routines can be a powerful way to mitigate existential and spiritual distress in a respectful, culturally attuned manner.

Building trust is also crucial, particularly for minority families, as cultural differences and past healthcare experiences may lead to distrust or reluctance to seek support. Culturally tailored care practices that honor the patient's cultural and spiritual values foster meaningful connections, creating a supportive environment where families and patients feel empowered. This foundation of trust and cultural respect enables families to engage in end-of-life planning with dignity and alignment to their beliefs, ensuring that care is both compassionate and personally relevant.

## The Cultural Formulation Interview (CFI) as a tool in dementia care

DSM-5 provides a valuable tool for enhancing cultural and spiritual understanding in treatment and care. It provides a structured approach, called the Cultural Formulation Interview (CFI), for early assessment of patients' backgrounds, beliefs, and values. By exploring cultural, spiritual, and existential dimensions, the CFI enables caregivers to gather essential information that supports person-centered and culturally attuned care. This framework encourages healthcare professionals to create individualized care plans that honor each patient's unique identity, fostering an environment of dignity, trust, and meaningful connection.

In dementia care, the CFI can be a practical guide to developing culturally sensitive approaches by enabling early engagement with patients and family members. This allows caregivers to gather insights that align care practices with patients' values and needs.

The CFI is designed to help clinicians explore the cultural dimensions of treatment and care by addressing how patients' cultural backgrounds influence their experiences, beliefs, and responses to illness. Here *culture* refers to "systems of knowledge, concepts, rules, and practices learned and transmitted across generations" (Aggarwal & Lewis-Fernández, 2015). The CFI helps bridge understanding between patients, caregivers, and healthcare providers by incorporating values, beliefs, and practices specific to the social groups to which patients belong, fostering collaborative insights into illness, treatment, and meaning-making.

The CFI can help create a comprehensive care plan that addresses medical needs as well as deeper cultural and spiritual dimensions by uncovering beliefs, traditions, and personal values that might otherwise remain hidden. Utilizing such tools in dementia care strengthens patient connection and identity, reinforcing dignity and respect as cognitive abilities decline.

## Structured interview

The *CFI consists of 16 structured questions* covering key areas such as beliefs about illness, support systems, and factors influencing self-coping. This approach is particularly useful in dementia care, where cultural beliefs about ageing, memory, and disease can vary significantly (DeSilva et al., 2018). The CFI is organized around four main areas that provide insights into patients' and families' cultural perspectives on dementia care:

*Cultural definition of the problem:* Focusing on understanding how the patient and family perceive the illness, questions may be formulated to ask to tell about any problems the patient has recently noticed. This can help caregivers recognize dementia symptoms within cultural contexts (Brooke et al., 2018).

*Cultural perceptions of cause, context, and support:* This area explores beliefs about the causes of dementia and sources of support. Adaptations may include questions like: "Who helps you feel better when confused or upset?" This is essential, as beliefs regarding causes, whether medical or spiritual, influence family involvement in care (Lai & Surood, 2013). Actual further questions are: "Why do you think this is happening to you?" and "What do you think are the causes of your problem?" Further, the patient is asked if there is any kind of support that alleviates his/her problem, like support from family or friends, and about stresses that the patients believe cause the problem to worsen, e.g. financial or family issues.

*Cultural factors affecting self-coping and past help-seeking:* Here, existing coping mechanisms and past help-seeking behaviors that are critical in dementia care are assessed. Rather than asking directly about personal coping, clinicians might ask family members about comforting activities that align with their loved one's cultural background. This method supports culturally aligned care practices, respecting traditional coping methods like religious support or rituals (Kenning et al., 2017). Further, the clinician asks about what the patient or relatives have done on their own to cope with the development of dementia. Actual questions relate to whether they have sought help from family, friends, or others, or help from alternative sources, such as healers or spiritual advisors.

*Cultural factors affecting clinical relationships:* The focus is on understanding expectations and building trust between patients, families, and providers. For instance, care providers might ask: "Are there things about your culture that are important for us to know as we care for your loved one?" This question is especially valuable for families who may feel distrustful due to previous healthcare experiences (Zubair, 2023). This can be followed by a question which specifically asks if there are any kinds of treatment he or she is looking for, and further, about what kind of care is seen as most important, as well as possible concerns about sharing information with healthcare providers because of one's cultural background.

Adapting the CFI for dementia care requires adjustments to ensure questions are clear and supportive for patients with cognitive impairment. When *simplifying language, incorporating family responses, and acknowledging cultural and religious beliefs,* the CFI can be a practical and helpful tool for existentially oriented dementia care, ensuring that the care plan is culturally relevant, respectful, and meaningful. By mapping cultural and religious preferences, the CFI can contribute to enhanced patient-centered care and foster a more inclusive, equitable healthcare experience for dementia patients (Brooke et al., 2018; Paralikar et al., 2020).

## Conclusion

Incorporating cultural, spiritual, and existential considerations into dementia care enhances the quality of life for individuals facing cognitive decline. By understanding and respecting cultural values and religious beliefs, caregivers can provide compassionate and personalized care that acknowledges each patient's unique identity. Family members play a crucial role in this process, preserving the patient's sense of continuity and belonging by sharing meaningful traditions and rituals. Such culturally sensitive practices not only help patients feel grounded but also support families in coping with the emotional and practical burdens of caregiving. Addressing biases, discrimination, and language barriers is essential for creating an inclusive and respectful care environment, especially for minority communities.

Tools like the Cultural Formulation Interview (CFI) help caregivers and healthcare professionals align care practices with the cultural and spiritual dimensions of patients' lives, promoting dignity and emotional comfort. Emotional regulation strategies are essential for both patients and caregivers to manage the emotional toll of cognitive decline. These strategies provide tools to navigate feelings such as grief, anxiety, frustration, and sadness, which are common for both parties in the caregiving journey. Combined with cultural rituals, further alleviate existential and spiritual distress, providing a familiar and supportive framework for patients and families alike. Ultimately, a cross-cultural approach to dementia care that includes family support, community resources, and culturally informed policy development is essential for meeting the complex needs of diverse populations. By recognizing the cultural, spiritual, and personal dimensions of dementia, caregivers can foster a compassionate, trust-based environment that respects each patient's journey, thereby enhancing both patient and caregiver well-being in meaningful and lasting ways.

## References

Aggarwal, N. K., & Lewis-Fernández, R. (2015). An introduction to the cultural formulation interview. *Focus, 13*(4), 426–431.

Brooke, J., Cronin, C., Stiell, M., & Ojo, O. (2018). The intersection of culture in the provision of dementia care: A systematic review. *Journal of Clinical Nursing, 27*(17–18), 3241–3253.

DeSilva, R., Aggarwal, N. K., & Lewis-Fernández, R. (2018). The DSM-5 Cultural Formulation Interview: Bridging barriers toward a clinically integrated cultural assessment in psychiatry. *Psychiatric Annals, 48*(3), 154–159.

Kenning, C., Daker-White, G., Blakemore, A., Panagioti, M., & Waheed, W. (2017). Barriers and facilitators in accessing dementia care by ethnic minority groups: A meta-synthesis of qualitative studies. *BMC Psychiatry, 17,* 1–13.

Kevern, P. (2015). The spirituality of people with late-stage dementia: A review of the research literature, a critical analysis and some implications for person-centered spirituality and dementia care. *Mental Health, Religion & Culture, 18*(9), 765–776.

Lai, D. W., & Surood, S. (2013). Effect of service barriers on health status of aging South Asian immigrants in Calgary, Canada. *Health & Social Work, 38*(1), 41–50.

Oyebode, J. R., & Parveen, S. (2019). Psychosocial interventions for people with dementia: An overview and commentary on recent developments. *Dementia, 18*(1), 8–35.

Paralikar, V. P., Deshmukh, A., & Weiss, M. G. (2020). Qualitative analysis of cultural formulation interview: Findings and implications for revising the outline for cultural formulation. *Transcultural Psychiatry, 57*(4), 525–541.

Robinson, C. A., Bottorff, J. L., Pesut, B., Oliffe, J. L., & Tomlinson, J. (2014). The male face of caregiving: A scoping review of men caring for a person with dementia. *American Journal of Men's Health, 8*(5), 409–426.

Sabat, S. R. (2001). The experience of' 'Alzheimer's disease: Life through atangled veil. *Psychiatric Bulletin, 27*(1), 39.

Swift, C. (2024). Spiritual care for people living with dementia. In Megan C. Best (ed.), *Spiritual Care in Palliative Care: What It Is and Why It Matters* (pp. 583–592). Cham: Springer Nature Switzerland.

Swinton, J. (2017). *Dementia: Living in the Memories of God.* Grand Rapids, MI: SCM Press.

Tsai, J. L., Koopmann-Holm, B., Miyazaki, M., & Ochs, C. (2013). The religious shaping of feeling. In R. F. Paloutzian & C. L. Park (eds.), *Handbook of the Psychology of Religion and Spirituality* (pp. 274–291). New York, NY: Guilford Press.

Yoon, K. H., Moon, Y. S., Lee, Y., Choi, S. H., Moon, S. Y., Seo, S. W.,..., & CARE (Caregivers of Alzheimer's Disease Research) Investigators. (2018). The moderating effect of religiosity on caregiving burden and depressive symptoms in caregivers of patients with dementia. *Aging & Mental Health, 22*(1), 141–147.

Zubair, M. (2023). Reframing' 'ethnicity'in dementia research: Reflections on current whiteness of research and the need for an anti-racist approach. In R. Ward & L. J. Sandberg (Eds.), *Critical Dementia Studies: An introduction* (pp. 83–99). London: Routledge.

# 13 The importance of an online discussion forum for caregivers in dementia care

*Hans Stifoss-Hanssen and Peter Kevern*

## Introduction

Being the closest relative of a person suffering from dementia, and a caregiver of that person, can amount to a crisis of a practical, emotional and not the least an existential nature (Large and Slinger, 2015). The caring role can be particularly challenging in the case of dementia because it changes the relationship between the carer and the person living with dementia. It typically develops gradually and persists for many years, so the existential 'identity' of both the person with dementia and their carer can be eroded (Smith et al., 2001; Jewell et al., 2017). The combination of mental and physical health issues and the complex nature of the challenges justifies the use of the term existential health to describe the situation: Existential health can be described as "the capacity to have faith in, to take care of, relate to, and experience meaning in life. It could encompass dimensions of inner peace and confidence" (Regeringen, 2024 web). The importance of existential health and the need to understand and support it are further discussed in the introductory chapter to this book.

To protect and restore their existential health in the face of these challenges, many carers express a desire to understand the 'meaning' of their experience or that of the person they are caring for. Although meaning-making is frequently linked to religious or spiritual beliefs and practices, efforts at making meaning can be recognized as a universal human tendency and capacity (Baumeister, 1992), and one of the key strategies of meaning-making is the development of narratives. These can be used to answer existential questions such as, "How did we get into this situation?" "What is this situation teaching us?" and "What is the purpose of this situation?". The use of self-narratives by people experiencing illness and existential challenge has been extensively studied (Frank, 1993, 2013). Existential meaning can be made or found even in situations of ongoing pain, and meaning in life can be expressed as micronarratives addressing particular situations, not necessarily linked to a global belief in the meaning of life (Baumeister, 1992). Indeed, personal meaning-making often takes the form of narrative fragments, symbols, images or ritual practices.

DOI: 10.4324/9781003517733-16

There is growing interest in the way narratives emerge and are presented in online conversations, since these give the opportunity for a group of people to share and to respond to each other without having to meet (Holtz, Kronberger and Wagner, 2012). An online forum is an interactive space in which contributions may be made in response to the contribution of others in 'real time', but also with longer delays between contributions: in some ways, it is like a face-to-face conversation, but in other ways it is like an exchange of correspondence.

## How we have studied the material

In this chapter, we will summarize some findings from our research study of the contributions to an online forum on spirituality and dementia that was hosted by the Alzheimers Society in 2013. The forum is a communication arena for personal carers, like spouses, sons and daughters, and other close relatives of persons with dementia. The discussion thread began with the question "… Are there any spiritual lessons to be gained through the journey of either the care giver or the victim?" and was active for about two weeks, resulting in a total of 64 contributions from 25 different people. In our research, we analyzed how participants "made meaning" by constructing narratives of their experience as carers. There is no space here to present a detailed account of our findings; but in what follows, we present two contrasting examples that illustrate some of the processes at work and discuss their relevance for the study of existential meaning-making.

## Case study A

One participant in the forum (A) presents himself as having authority to speak and something to say, on the basis of his experiences and achievements over a long and varied life. His story starts with a short summary and then stretches over five long contributions which unfold in a theatrical manner. A tells about a deprived childhood which built character and survival skills. He then tells about 'Salvation' in meeting his wife, followed by national and international success: he says he was able to retire at 64. Then, his wife's dementia and his experience of nursing her, which was a "privilege, an honour, humbling experience and the most rewarding time" of his life. He thanks God for providing him with the strength to care for her to the end.

A's reflection on his life culminates in the privilege of caring for his wife, and an opening to the future: his harsh upbringing and deprived childhood turned out to have been ordained to prepare and strengthen him for the challenge of caring for his wife, which he now believes to have been the whole purpose of his life. A mainly uses the online forum as a platform on which to develop and present his story, which is to display the attributes of his wife, and

his continued love for her: "... she was my salvation and still inspires me...".
Thus, the purpose of his contribution is not so much to contribute to an answer
to the question of meaning for carers in general as to bear witness to his wife
and to the way the meaningfulness of his own life emerges in a continuous,
integrated narrative.

*Case study D*

Another participant (D) defines her religious position carefully, as an atheist
gaining new spiritual insights into life. She is also the only contributor who
cites her academic background (a psychology degree). These two elements
are central to D's overall approach, because she is about to present a summary
of key ideas from Deepak Chopra which could be 'fringe' Psychology and/or
'alternative Religion', so they serve as warrants of her credibility as a witness
to them.

   The overall story of D is of her finding enlightenment through the spiritual
challenge of dementia. In her childhood, she says, "The tentacles of religion
(NOT spirituality) crushed any budding spirituality". But in her role as carer,
everything that she assumed "vanished under the onslaught of Dementia".
This process led her to an inner peace in which she found healing. So the
account of her journey ends with the conclusion that there is a meaning in
"walking the Dementia Journey".

   The vehicle for this transformation is a schema in Deepak Chopra's book,
*How to know God* (Chopra, 2007). This provides a framework for her own
account of transformation. She maintains that her experience of caring for
somebody with Alzheimer's Disease has impelled her to "develop areas of
my brain that were dormant". For this she is grateful, as the "Alzheimer's
Onslaught" has exposed to her inner spiritual resources. If this is understood
as a testimony, the role of the audience is to serve as witnesses to validate it,
although unlike an evangelistic testimony, D does not seem to want to con-
vince others that this is the only way.

   D is making an argument for viewing her own (and by extension, others') experience of caring for someone with dementia as a process of spiritual
growth and transformation. D demonstrates how she has grown spiritually:
she has been forced to 'make meaning' in response to the challenging situation and has found that there were sources of help and inspiration. In a broader
sense, she may be read as testifying that there is a spirituality beyond inherited
religion, attainable through growth and suffering, and this provides her with
an account of the meaningfulness of her carer experience.

*Other case study material*

The participants differed widely in their contributions and used the forum
in different ways to support their meaning-making activity. They positioned
themselves in diverse ways in relation to other contributors, and in some cases

described their own position and background with some care. These positioning moves were themselves part of meaning-making, as contributors aligned with or (less often) challenged the interpretations of others on the forum. In this way, the audience became implicitly present in each contributor's story.

Some stories were quite lengthy and were supplemented with additional contributions during the course of the exchange, but in one instance, the focus was directed towards his/her spiritual/religious learning outcome – typically related to alternative or idiosyncratic spirituality. Disappointment with established religion was characteristic.

As in the case of A, several posters interacted explicitly with other contributors, shaping their story in relationship and response to previous statements. Whereas meaning-making can be seen as the chief purpose of the stories that were told, responding to the challenge made by the initial contributor seeking: "...thoughts which lend a spiritual perspective to going through dementia", meaning is shaped differently by the contributors. Some narrated their "the dementia journey" as a tragedy, but some kind of constructive purpose of the contributions was common, from the personal witness to having experienced meaningfulness in the experience, to the more proactive recommendation of specific existential alternatives.

### Some reflections on the cases, and what to learn

Although all participants claim their primary authority to speak from their experience of dementia, this is shaped and supported in different ways: by life story, by religious belief, by the implied presence of others, and by academic and literary contributions.

Online contributions to a discussion group are produced and staged in a characteristic way. This activity helps make sense of the complexity of human lives, for example, when reflecting on the experience of caring for somebody with dementia.

We have also observed a common, collaborative attempt among the participants to find meaning. We call this a dimension of **internarrativity**, it shows itself in the ways the participants recognize, support and occasionally contradict or correct each other. This may be understood as a common effort to place narratives alongside, giving a complex, but fascinating account of the lives of the carers. The contributions represent construction of meaning in reflection upon experience. The act of storytelling is an effort at making sense, combatting chaos, tolerating ambiguity. The telling of stories implies arranging selected moments from the mess in some order and making it less painful.

Meaning-making narratives are constructively created together with other people. Consequently, the narratives may be not just for the benefit of the narrator, but of others, in a community. In the social context, the different persons' narratives are woven together, and 'feed' each other. This amounts to a dimension of internarrativity that is often overlooked. What is noteworthy is that we have arrived at this understanding of existential meaning-making not from a therapeutic perspective but by listening to the stories: the activity of narrative meaning-making imposes its own productive logic on the situation. According to V DeMarinis, existential health is a crucial dimension of public mental health, and it is closely linked to the experience of modern life as being unstable and fragmented (DeMarinis, 2003). Persons with dementia and their family carers are vulnerable to these risk factors in modern life, since a major share of caring practices take place within private homes and in the voluntary sector. Persons with dementia and their carers do have the opportunity to maintain some degree of good existential health, but that requires good strategies for meaning-making. And making meaning – or experiencing meaning – is very often supported and strengthened through telling and sharing of narratives.

## References

Baumeister, R.F. (1992) 'Neglected aspects of self-theory: Motivation, interpersonal aspects, culture, escape, and existential value', *Psychological Inquiry*, 3(1), pp. 21–25.
Chopra, D (2007) *How to know God: The soul's journey into the mystery of mysteries.* New York: Harmony.
DeMarinis V. (2003). *Pastoral care, existential health, and existential epidemiology.* Stockholm: Verbum.
Frank, A.W. (1993) 'The rhetoric of self-change : Illness experience as narrative', *Sociological Quarterly*, 34(1), pp. 39–52.
Frank, A.W. (2013) *The wounded storyteller: Body, illness, and ethics.* Chicago: University of Chicago Press.
Holtz, P., Kronberger, N. and Wagner, W. (2012) 'Analyzing Internet forums a practical guide', *Journal of Media Psychology*, 24(2), pp. 55–66. Available at: https://doi.org/10.1027/1864-1105/a000062.
Jewell, A. et al. (2017) 'The loneliness of the long-distance carer: The experience of primary carers of loved-ones with dementia', *Rural Theology*, 15(2), pp. 97–112. Available at: https://doi.org/10.1080/14704994.2017.1373473.
Large, S. and Slinger, R. (2015) 'Grief in caregivers of persons with Alzheimer's disease and related dementia: A qualitative synthesis', *Dementia*, 14(2), pp. 164–183. Available at: https://doi.org/10.1177/1471301213494511.
Regeringen (2024) https://www.regeringen.se/pressmeddelanden/2024/04/uppdrag-for-att-utveckla-arbetet-med-existentiell-halsa-i-folkhalsopolitiken/
Smith, A.L. et al. (2001) 'Caregiver needs: A qualitative exploration', *Clinical Gerontologist*, 24(1/2), pp. 3–26. Available at: https://doi.org/10.1300/J018v24n01_02.

# 14 The presence of the past

## Existential dementia care in a life tapestry perspective

*Lars Johan Danbolt*

We can look at life as a line, but also as a tapestry. These metaphors can go well together, but also offer different perspectives. The line metaphor helps us recognize chronology and see life events in sequence. Perhaps we also recognize the dynamics of what leads to what in our life history as well as where unexpected incidents fracture or mess up our lives for a period. The tapestry metaphor, however, shows a picture with interwoven elements that are simultaneously present. A life tapestry can be vast, sometimes requiring distance to see the whole, while at other times, we need to focus on smaller sections. As Lakoff and Johnson (2008) state, we live by our metaphors. In professional life, we also work by our metaphors. It is, of course, not given that we all live or work by the same kind of metaphors, and that might be an important issue in the relationship between patient and professional in dementia care where the subject-to-subject relationship is crucial.

In this chapter, we draw on the life tapestry metaphor to reflect some of the themes mentioned in this book. We ask: Do people with dementia more or less leave the present to live in the past? Or is it more likely to think that they integrate their past into their experience of the present?

## Meaning as an integrated life endeavor

Of course, interest in one's past is not reserved for people with dementia. Remembering past experiences and constructing life narratives is a rather common human experience, especially as we age (Vissers et al., 2024). Through our life-narratives in mature age, we make the past present, giving our experiences, relationships, and episodes meaning. Life stories across lifespan have the potential to make our experiences coherent and directed, as well as significant and belonging, which is the content of the experience of life as meaningful (Schnell, 2021).

Life cycle researcher Erikson (Erikson & Erikson, 1998) proposed that in mature age (65+), the main mental conflict is between ego integrity and despair, and that important events in this age relate to reflections on life, for many generating wisdom. People with dementia may have reduced capacity

DOI: 10.4324/9781003517733-17

to reflect on their life history due to cognitive impairment. Still there are examples of how people with dementia draw meaning from their past experiences and make them significant for their present sense of meaning in life. Cases described by Nylund and Feiring in Chapter 11 can illustrate this. For example, Daisy, a nursing home resident with severe dementia, often referred back to her family and other important relationships when telling about meaning in life. Her timeline was dissolved, as Nylund and Feiring noted, with the past woven into her present experience of meaning. Another resident, Oscar, mentioned that he had learned valuable lessons from his grandparents, which he passed on to his grandchildren. For him, meaning was linked to his role as someone who received something valuable and passed it on to future generations—a source of meaning that Erikson described as generativity (Schnell, 2021). Chapter 11 also gives an example of not being able to experience these dynamics. Jenny, who was in an early stage of dementia, longed for her home and family, contrasting it with her nursing home experiences. She perceived the other residents, who sat doing nothing, as passive and sick, something she feared becoming herself.

## Talking about experiences of meaning

Probably, many working in person-centered dementia care may recognize that yes; it is possible to talk about meaning in life, sources of meaning and perhaps crises of meaning. But it also happens that communication about the existential experiences of being *me* in *my* life as it is at the moment, fades into silence if this is not being actively followed up in the dialogue between the person living with dementia and a professional or family-related caregiver.

When asked about meaning in life, individuals with dementia may recall events from decades ago, making them valid in the current moment of the conversation. A person can tell about how her life is significant to others and refer to her role as a mother or wife or business partner, nurse or teacher a long time ago, and the distinction between *had* and *has* significance is blurred. If we orient ourselves by a line metaphor, this is confusing, and we often feel the urge to reorient the other to a here and now perspective. The tapestry metaphor, however, might help us see life as a whole picture, as well as to see our role as care personnel to assist the other person in weaving his or her life tapestry. The tapestry is not a finished piece of work; it is continually being woven as it is presented. And the weaver is not only the person with dementia, but also the one or ones talking with her or him. It is a dialogical project between subjects, and along with the development of the illness, the narrative, as well as the self of the person living with dementia become increasingly relational.

## Dialogical relationships

People with dementia often struggle to express themselves, with fragmented memories and difficulty maintaining focus on their own. This makes relational dialogue important. In this context, "dialogue" refers to a conversation with certain qualities: clarity, honesty, and without hidden agendas that could arouse suspicion. Dialogue seeks to enhance equality, uncover power asymmetry, biases and misunderstandings, avoid infantilization and stigma, and promote reciprocity and respect for differences. Through dialogue, we pay attention to the vague and heterogeneous, as well as to contradictions and resistance. A life tapestry is never clear and easy to interpret. It will be filled with contradictions and tensions, ugliness and frustration, light and dark colors, and sometimes blurred and confusing sections. It is the owner of the tapestry's privilege to decide where the attention should be drawn in the large picture. In that way dialogue is a way of exploring meaning and together weave fragments of the life tapestry the person with dementia can live by.

Dialogues are social intersubjective activities that enhance a sense of togetherness. Existential health is a first-person experience. It is *I* who live *my* life. The suffering, diagnoses, and illnesses are *mine*, as are hope, belief, and the life tapestry. Existential health opposes all kinds of objectifications. People are 'I' and not 'it'. This emphasis is reflected in the language of person-centered care, such as using 'person living with dementia' instead of 'demented person'. When it comes to people with severe dementia, the 'I' is very dependent on a 'we', which also to some degree is the case for all of us. As Brown states, "Dementia reminds us that when we ask where value lies in people, we also need to recognize that it lies *between* people, lodged within their attachments" (Brown, 2017, page 1010). That does not mean that the 'I' is dissolved into a 'we'-unity, but rather that individuals with dementia interact with others within a dynamic of togetherness.

Cognitive impairment is a collective experience, and not just an individual state. In dialogue, both cognition and memory are present. Professional caregivers or family members lend cognition and memory to the person with dementia, making these resources available for the person with cognitive impairment. In this way, dialogue constitutes a small social group where the person with dementia is continually re-membered as a human being, belonging in communities and re-equipped with 'shuttle and tread' and assisted in 'weaving' on his or her life tapestry.

## Artifacts and symbols bridging time and space

When dealing with difficulties from the past, pictures and other artefacts charged with memory and meaning can be valuable, as well as symbols and rituals. Sometimes communication goes beyond words, and nonverbal interactions can function better. A gentle touch, a smile, and a nod, pointing at a picture or showing or demonstrating something, walking together, or listening to music, singing or simply be silent together, can be experienced as significant sense of togetherness. Chapter 5 provides good examples of this.

Further, use of symbols and rituals can be a way to communicate. Symbols— items charged with personal or cultural meaning—help bridge spans of time and space. For instance, a candle lit in a church as a symbol of hope can be mirrored by a candle on a kitchen table, reminding someone of that hope. Symbols are often part of rituals, which can be seen as symbolic activities that create meaning (Danbolt & Stifoss-Hanssen, 2017). Symbols and rituals serve as a 'third element' that both participants in a dialogue relate to, fostering a sense of togetherness. Together we seek to reconcile and find peace and hope. Both symbols and rituals will normally be sensitive to cultural and religious traditions, which, of course, also have to be respected in dialogue between a person with dementia and a care person.

Some of the same dynamics can be seen by using the SoMe Card method as described in Chapter 10. The cards also represent a 'third element' that can facilitate dialogue about meaning and existential issues when words are missing. The cards are visual statements that both dialogue partners can relate to, dismiss, feel angry about, or feel drawn toward, opening for something regarded as important in the situation.

## Reconciling the past

Life threads are often complex in older adults, and many may feel the need to reconcile the past and accept their lives (Vissers et al., 2024). The stress from what happened in the past affects the present, and for many there is a desire to reconcile something that cannot be changed. However, the narrative about difficult episodes and how they are dealt with and perhaps reconciled can be integrated in present life in meaningful ways. For people living with cognitive impairments and memory loss, reflection is a challenging task and the support from others in dialogue is crucial.

Reconciliation of the past often goes hand in hand with the need for a fulfilled purpose of life. For many elderly people this relates to what Erikson described as the main mental conflict in mature age; ego integrity versus despair and the urge to reflect upon one's life to accept, reconcile, and integrate a sense of meaningfulness. For people with cognitive deficits and memory loss, the endeavor of life history reflections is more or less out of range, but fragments, episodes, and bodily procedural memories stimulated by emotions, artefacts, traditions, rituals, places, and other reminiscent experiences are active.

## Continuation and coherence

Continuation, the sense of being in line with what was considered valuable earlier in life, is a dimension in meaningfulness that is found to be prominent in late life (Vissers et al., 2024). Perhaps there is a sense of 'ageless self' as Kaufman (1986) called it some decades ago. This concept has later been criticized for romanticizing ageing (Luborsky, 2023), and our selves are probably relative to ageing as is the case for our entire biopsychosocial constitution.

Nevertheless, despite this process of ageing there seem to be a continuation from what was considered meaningful before the onset of severe illness and present life (Haug et al., 2016).

However, self is not necessarily a stable construct, but something that is constantly coming into being (Brown, 2017). For people living with dementia in late stages, the self can be fragmented with reduction or loss of memory and language. The self increasingly dwells in the relationship between the people as a collective responsibility, making persons living with dementia dependent on the relational sustainability of their surroundings. See more about this in Chapter 3.

The impact of dementia on self and identity is a big discussion. A systematic review by Caddell and Clare (2010) found that there is some evidence for persistence of self also in later stages of dementia. It is also found that in persons living with Alzheimer's disease the memory of personal experiences (autobiographical memory), which is important for how we define ourselves and construct meaningful life stories, can be declined, leading to an impaired sense of identity and self (El Haj et al., 2015). However, the definition of self is another big discussion. What seems to be important is the relational approach to dementia care.

Coherence and continuation are important dimensions of meaningfulness among elderly people generally. Schnell found that independent of age violation of one's sense of coherence and continuity can result in a crisis of meaning, an intrusive experience of life as empty, meaningless, and not worth living (Schnell, 2009). We do not know whether the onset and progression of dementia affect the experience of crises of meaning. Does dementia cause such crises, or does the cognitive decline diminish the person's ability to recognize them, letting the sense of meaninglessness—as well as perhaps meaningfulness—fade beyond consciousness?

There is no clear answer to that, but it is reason to believe that there are continuities through life regarding experiences of meaningfulness and crises of meaning, as well as sources of meaning. It is likely to assume that the complexity of good and bad life trajectories is present and not beyond consciousness, whatever that means, but ineffable and hard to express when the usual bearings of cognition and memory are about to dissolve. Thus, a working-model in the care for people with dementia should include an awareness and sensitivity to the vague and unsaid between the expressions in the dialogue, sensing the heterogeneous and contradictory, and the fluctuations in moods and emotions (cf. Chapter 9).

## Existentially healthy care

For many people with dementia, there is a tension between sense of belonging and sense of alienation. Nursing home residents may feel well cared for, but studies also show that they can experience loneliness, lack of relationships, and loss of autonomy and privacy (Ericson-Lidman, 2019). Disorientation, often a result of dementia, further contributes to feelings of existential isolation and alienation, as well as hopelessness and helplessness (Dzwiza-Ohlsen, 2022). Rational and relational capacity of people with dementia decline over time, making them increasingly dependent on others. It has been debated whether the individual "I" can be absorbed into a collective "we." Critics of that idea argue that persons with dementia risk being dissolved into an undifferentiated unity (Dzwiza-Ohlsen, 2022). In existentially oriented dementia care, it is important to maintain the individuality of the person—their history, culture, beliefs, and preferences are theirs. Dementia does not dissolve these aspects but rather makes the person's sense of self more dependent on a supportive, relational environment. In other words, existential health in people with dementia is to a significant extent a matter of existentially healthy care.

## Some recommendations

- As a dialogue partner with persons living with dementia, equip yourself with well-functioning metaphors—metaphors we can work by. Making life tapestry together might be one.
- Explore the significance of past experiences for meaning in the moment you talk.
- Lend cognitive capacity to the dialogue to keep focus.
- Be open for use of artefacts, symbols, and rituals, but never intrusive and with awareness for timing.

## References

Brown, J. (2017). Self and identity over time: Dementia. *Journal of Evaluation in Clinical Practice, 23*(5), 1006–1012.
Caddell, L. S., & Clare, L. (2010). The impact of dementia on self and identity: A systematic review. *Clinical Psychology Review, 30*(1), 113–126.
Danbolt, L. J., & Stifoss-Hanssen, H. (2017). Ritual and recovery: Traditions in disaster ritualizing. *Dialog, 56*(4), 352–360.
Dzwiza-Ohlsen, E. N. (2022). Going Home Alone? – On Disorientation, Homelessness, and We-Identity in Alzheimer's Dementia. *Methodo, Special Issue: Familiarity and Togetherness*, 1–24.
El Haj, M., Antoine, P., Nandrino, J. L., & Kapogiannis, D. (2015). Autobiographical memory decline in Alzheimer's disease, a theoretical and clinical overview. *Ageing Research Reviews, 23*, 183–192.
Erikson, E. H., & Erikson, J. M. (1998). *The life cycle completed (extended version).* WW Norton & Company. New York.
Ericson-Lidman, E. (2019). Struggling between a sense of belonging and a sense of alienation: Residents' experiences of living in a residential care facility for older people in Sweden. *Nordic Journal of Nursing Research, 39*(3), 143–151.

Haug, S. H. K., Danbolt, L. J., Kvigne, K., & DeMarinis, V. (2016). Older people with incurable cancer: Existential meaning-making from a life-span perspective. *Palliative & Supportive Care, 14*(1), 20–32.

Kaufman, S. R. (1986). *The ageless self: Sources of meaning in late life.* University of Wisconsin Press.

Lakoff, G., & Johnson, M. (2008). *Metaphors we live by.* University of Chicago Press.

Luborsky, M. (2023). The ageless self: A relic or the reliquary? *Anthropology & Aging, 44*(1), 92–101.

Schnell, T. (2009). The Sources of Meaning and Meaning in Life Questionnaire (SoMe): Relations to demographics and well-being. *The Journal of Positive Psychology, 4*(6), 483–499.

Schnell, T. (2021). *The psychology of meaning in life.* Routledge. New York.

Vissers, J., Peltomäki, I., Duppen, D., Haugan, G., Larsson, H., Saarelainen, S. M., & Dezutter, J. (2024). Meaning in late life: A scoping review. *Journal of Happiness Studies, 25*(1), 21.

# Forgotten but not disappeared

Forgotten
but not disappeared
merely hidden
in everyday stream

We cannot remember
accomplishments many
they fade and resurface
in every night's dream

Memories
missing
we still are here
conspicuously absent
and still nearby
as everything
changing
remains

That which escapes us
has not lost its meaning
rather like pointers
showing the way

from past to present
and further ahead
we cannot detect it
but know all the same

Memories
missing

DOI: 10.4324/9781003517733-18

we still are here
silently present
in every touch
as everything
changing
remains

Memories lost
are still ours to keep
we continuously dwell there
from daybreak to dusk

Forgotten
but not disappeared
merely concealed
under heaven's dome

If no one can force
time to its knees
the wings of the wind
will still carry us here
to this place
where we'll always
remain
                    Sturla J. Stålsett

# Index

meaning in life as 14; health *see* existential health; paradoxes of 12–13; philosophy 5, 6; psychology 5, 6; psychotherapy 7; suffering 15; themes, in nursing homes *see* persons with dementia; threats 65; well-being 4, 23, 25, 26
existential health 3, 8, 21–23, 25, 67, 104, 108, 111; in dementia 9–10, 13–14; healthcare professionals, role of 93–94; healthy care 113–114; matters 87; person-centered care and *see* person-centered care; and persons with dementia *see* persons with dementia; social nature of 9–10
existentially healthy care 113–114
existential philosophy 5, 12; "dizziness of freedom" 15
expressions: creative expression 73; in dialogue 113; emotional expression 69; of existential crisis 40; of life on Earth 8; of meaning in life 42, 92; qualities and 6–7; of significance 30

families: cultural perspectives, on dementia care 101; in dementia care 96
fear of dementia 20–21; "dying again, and again, and again" 24–27; hypercognitive society 21–22; person as 'living dead' 23–24; social self 22–23
Food and Drug Administration (FDA) 58
frontotemporal dementia (FTD) 56, 70, 76; frontotemporal lobe dementia 66–67; behavioral variant (bvFTD) patients 70

gender 33; dynamics 97; issues 97–98; roles 35, 98

health 3–4; biopsychosocial model of 4, 13, 14, 49; dimensions of 7–9; environmental health 8; existential health *see* existential health; health-as-function 10; mental health 7; psychological health 7; social health 7, 8
*Horizontal Selftranscendence*, sources of meaning 82
humanism/humanistic: disciplines 5; perspective in medicine 4; psychology 5
'hypercognitive' society 21–22

identity 13, 38, 51, 76, 89; constructs of 22; core of 96; cultural identity 34, 99; emotions in 71; existential identity 104; loss of 33; and meaning 73; person's sense of 50, 69, 74; sense of 113
"I-It" meeting 47, 51
integrated model of health 4; *see also* biopsychosocial model
internarrativity 107
"I-Thou" meeting 47, 52, 74

*Lancet Commision of the dementia prevention, intervention, and care (2024)* 57
language: barriers 98; level, of dementia 24
Lewy body dementia (LBD) 56, 59, 70, 76
life story narrative movement, in dementia care 86
life tapestry, existential dementia care: artifacts and symbols 111–112; continuation and coherence 112–113; dialogical relationships 110–111; existentially healthy care 113–114; experiences of meaning 110; meaning, as integrated life endeavor 109–110; reconciliation of the past 112
loneliness 29, 32, 35, 64, 81, 92, 113
long-term care nursing homes 89–90

malignant social psychology 23, 51
Meaning and Purpose Scales (MAPS) 90
meaningfulness 14, 106, 109–110; and crisis of meaning 85; dimensions of existential health 47, 53, 112–113; existential concept of meaning in life 49–51; experience of 39, 107; as motivator and buffer 17; sense of 18; and sources of meaning 90
meaning in life 5, 6, 37–38, 41–42, 56, 82–84, 93; daily life and 64; existential concept of 49–51; as existential foundation 14; experience of 90; mental and physical health 17; perception of 66; persons' religious references and 57; quality of life and 9, 48; residents' experience of 52–53; sense of 62, 110
meaning-making narratives 107
Mediterranean diet 58

For Product Safety Concerns and Information please contact our EU
representative  GPSR@taylorandfrancis.com
Taylor & Francis Verlag GmbH, Kaufingerstraße 24, 80331 München, Germany